SPARTAN
WARRIOR WORKOUT

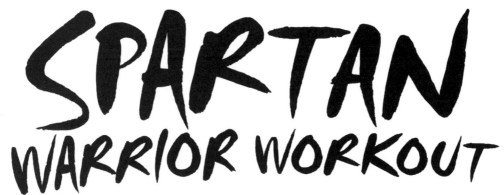

SPARTAN
WARRIOR WORKOUT

GET ACTION-MOVIE RIPPED IN **30** DAYS

DAVE RANDOLPH

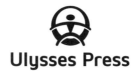

Ulysses Press

Published in the United States by
Ulysses Press
P.O. Box 3440
Berkeley, CA 94703
www.ulyssespress.com

ISBN: 978-1-56975-791-8
Library of Congress Control Number 2009943778

Printed in Canada by Webcom

10 9 8 7 6 5 4 3 2

Acquisitions: Keith Riegert
Managing editor: Claire Chun
Editor: Lily Chou
Proofreader: Lauren Harrison
Production: Judith Metzener, Abigail Reser
Index: Sayre Van Young
Cover design: what!design @ whatweb.com
Cover photograph: © istockphoto.com/Damir Spanic
Interior photographs: © Rapt Productions except on page 9: © shutterstock.com/
    photobank.kiev.ua; page 12: © shutterstock.com/Pavel Ignatov; pages 13 & 16:
    © shutterstock.com/Robyn Mackenzie; page 17: © shutterstock.com/Jerry
    Horbert; pages 49 (bottom), 52, 89 (bottom), 99, 110, 112 (top), 113, 114 (top),
    115, 146 © Jessica Power
Models: Dave Randolph, Rance Hayes, Meredith Miller, Jeff Vick, Julie Boggess

Distributed by Publishers Group West

Please Note
This book has been written and published strictly for informational purposes, and in no way should be used as a substitute for actual instruction with qualified professionals. The author and publisher are providing you with information in this work so that you can have the knowledge and can choose, at your own risk, to act on that knowledge. The author and publisher also urge all readers to be aware of their health status and to consult health care professionals before beginning any health program.

Contents

PART 4: *Appendix*

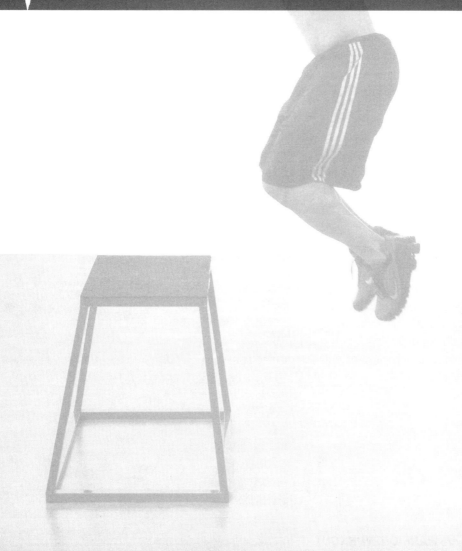

PART 1

Getting Started

Introduction

You might've seen the movie *300* when it came out in 2007. The film is a screen adaptation of a graphic novel that was based upon the Battle of Thermopylae in August or September of 480 B.C., as chronicled by the Greek historian Herodotus. During the battle, Greece was invaded by the Persians, who were led by their king Xerxes and his armies, which numbered in the millions. At the time, Greece was not a unified country but many city-states, each led by their own ruler. The Spartan army was the main force and was led by King Leonidas I. He and 300 of his royal guard, along with men from several other city-states, built an army of about 7,000 warriors to hold off the overwhelming Persian army.

The Spartans from the city-state of ancient Greece have been known through the ages as a very fierce band of people. The men were raised from birth to be self-sufficient and expert fighters. They learned sword-play, hand-to-hand fighting, and the use of the bow and spear from a very early age. They trained hard so that they would be victorious on the field of battle. Modern historians believe the Spartans were very lean and athletic due in part to their warrior life-style and the scarcity of food. The Spartans had to learn to survive long periods with little or no food while continually training or fighting.

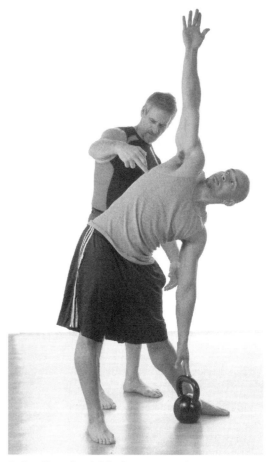

In order for the film's actors to look like the characters they portrayed, director Zach Snyder hired well-known fitness expert and climber Mark Twight to whip the cast into shape. Twight crafted an intense, five-month training program that not only chiseled the actors but also enabled them to handle the rigors of filming the fight scenes, which often took hours.

If you think you already have what it takes to be a Spartan, take the challenge on page 7 and go from there. What if you can't do a perfect pull-up or push-up, or you're just getting back on the fitness track? No problem. *Spartan Warrior Workout* details the exercises that make up the *300* workout and provides programs to make you stronger, faster and more powerful while helping you burn off unwanted fat.

Author Dave Randolph gives some pointers.

The Spartan Warrior Workout

Training methods such as bodybuilding or powerlifting create, in most people, bulky, non-functional muscles rather than lean, lithe, coordinated and healthy bodies that should be our ideal. Big, bulky muscles are not a survival trait. They require a lot more energy to maintain and are, in most cases, not functional, slow you down and can limit your range of motion—all of which can get you killed in the field of battle. Mark Twight's training program utilized a wide variety of equipment and lots of bodyweight exercises (calisthenics), focusing on exercises that require full-body control, coordination and awareness, to get the cast ripped while retaining their athletic build. High-intensity interval training (HIIT) and functional whole-body movements prevented his charges from getting big and bulky.

Using barbells, kettlebells, calisthenics (pull-ups and push-ups) and strongman exercises (e.g., heavy tire flipping, sled pulling and pushing), Twight pushed the actors hard for one to two hours every day for four months before filming began and they continued to train during the filming. His workouts were very intense and never done more than once. This made them physically challenging since the actors never knew in advance what they'd be doing; their bodies were always kept guessing. The arduous workouts also forced the actors and crew to develop the warrior mindset—if you give up, quit or don't put forth maximum effort, you will die. The end result of all this hard work was a group of actors and crew that was extremely fit and mentally tough and looked like what we think the Spartans probably did, based upon the many Greek and Roman statues from that era.

One of the workouts the actors did came to be known as the "300 Workout." It was designed to see how far the actors had come in their conditioning and strength training. Basically, the workout taxes the body's major muscle groups and focuses on pulling and pushing movements in the horizontal and vertical planes. While this workout was one of many, it was actually a test that Twight put the top performers through. The workout consisted of:

- 25 dead-hang pull-ups
- 50 deadlifts
- 50 push-ups
- 50 box jumps
- 50 floor wipers
- 50 kettlebell dead clean and press (25 per side)
- 25 dead-hang pull-ups

These were to be done as quickly as possible, which meant little to no rest during the workout. One actor from the film, Andrew Pleavin, completed the workout in 18 minutes, 11 seconds—a grueling pace!

Training Overview

Some fitness experts break down and design training programs based on whether a movement is a vertical push like a squat (pushing up from the floor), a vertical pull like a pull-up, a horizontal push like a push-up/bench press, or a horizontal pull like a rowing machine. In addition, the movements can be further subdivided into upper and lower body.

- Upper body vertical pull—pull-up
- Upper body vertical push—the press
- Lower body vertical pull—deadlift or kettlebell clean
- Lower body vertical push—squat
- Upper body horizontal pull—rowing machine
- Upper body horizontal push—push-up or bench press
- Lower body horizontal pull—hamstring curl on a machine

Many times trainers try to combine movements from all these categories into a workout. Others may focus on only one or two elements, depending on their clients' goals.

Some exercises, especially kettlebell movements or the Olympic lifts, have many of these elements in them. The dead clean is one example. It's a vertical pull from the floor, but there's actually a squat component with an explosive upward extension of the hips, knees and, in some cases, ankle. The minor element is an upper body pull with the trapezius, but that's about 10 percent of the overall movement.

Twight's workout incorporated movements in these different planes to stress the body in ways that are natural, using the whole body to generate force rather than isolating body parts like bodybuilders do. Because the actors were trying to get lean and weren't training for a specific task like that of a sport, Twight's training programs always changed, never letting the body adapt to any one thing but instead preparing the body for whatever was thrown at it. This is known as General Physical Preparedness, or GPP, in the fitness industry; you can think of it as being "in shape."

In reality, GPP is merely a base upon which an athlete would build the skills necessary for his/her specific sport. For example, a fighter would build up his GPP and, as his base improved, his training would concentrate more on the techniques of punching, kicking or grappling. Football players build their GPP before the season starts; as the start of the season nears, they focus more on honing the skills needed to be the best they can at their position. We'll talk more about GPP on page 111. The next step after GPP is known as sport-specific preparation, or SPP; this is where the athlete practices specific skills to master a sport or game.

THE EXERCISES

Throughout this book you'll learn six specific exercises that are done in this workout: pull-up, deadlift, push-up, box jump, floor wiper, and dead clean and press. You'll also learn variations of the main movements and a number of assistance exercises that augment the primary movements. For example, the incline push-up is a push-up variation, while the bench press is an assistance exercise to the push-up. For those of you who need some extra

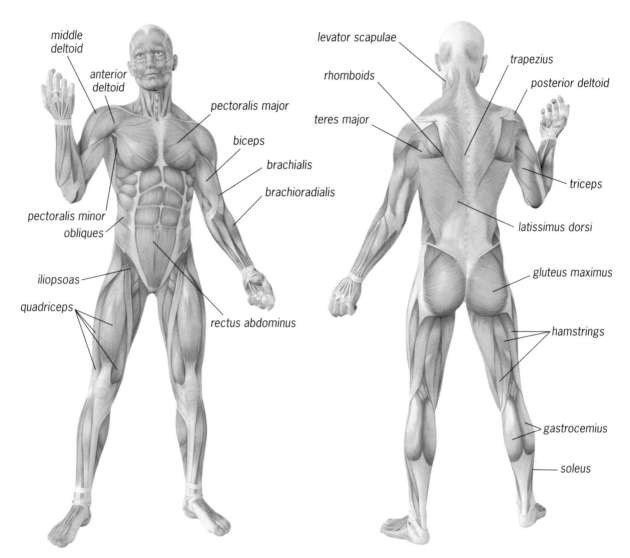

middle
deltoid

anterior
deltoid

pectoralis major

biceps

brachialis

brachioradialis

pectoralis minor

obliques

iliopsoas

quadriceps

rectus abdominus

levator scapulae

rhomboids

teres major

trapezius

posterior deltoid

triceps

latissimus dorsi

gluteus maximus

hamstrings

gastrocemius

soleus

attention (maybe you're barely able to do a push-up or unable to do any pull-ups), we've designed the programs so that you'll be doing 5 to 10 or more without a break in no time.

At the end of this program, which may take you several cycles to really get down, you'll have forged your body into a lean, statuesque figure and made yourself mentally tough, able to withstand any mental stress life may throw at you.

Pull-ups

Pull-ups are a vertical pulling movement. When done properly, the entire core (meaning the abs and back) is involved, as are the *gluteus maximus* and *hamstrings*. Creating tension throughout the body recruits more muscle fibers, which makes you stronger. This is known as the principle of hyperirradiation (according to Pavel Tsatsouline in *Power to the People!: Russian Strength Training Secrets for Every American*) and should be applied to most exercises, especially when lifting heavy weight. For the best results, the Spartan Warrior Workout uses "dead-hang" pull-ups, not kipping pull-ups. There should be little to no swing at the bottom; each rep should stop and start from a dead stop. Kipping is cheating.

The primary muscles worked by the pull-up are the *latissimus dorsi* (lats). Other muscles involved (called synergists) are the *brachialis, brachioradialis, teres major, posterior deltoid, rhomboids, levator scapulae*, and the lower and middle portions of the *trapezius* (most people only think of the upper traps when talking about them). All of those, with the exception of the brachialis and brachioradialis, are on the back. On the front of the body, the *pectoralis major* (sternal head) and *pectoralis minor* are both involved in pull-ups.

Deadlifts

Deadlifts are a classic barbell exercise and possibly the most "functional" lift, too. Top deadlifters have pulled over 1,000 pounds, or a half-ton, from the floor. The movement is primarily a lower body pull, but because the hands are the end link in the chain of muscles, the whole body must work in unison. The legs drive the hips forward and the torso rises, while all the while the arms are straight and all the force is put into the bar through the hands. In most people, the grip is the weakest link, and powerlifters routinely do supplemental grip work to strengthen their hands.

The prime movers are the *gluteus maximus* (glutes), *hamstrings* and the muscles of the entire *back* (including the trapezius, latissimus dorsi and rhomboids); the *calves*, hamstrings, glutes and lower back are known as the posterior chain. The *deltoids* are also heavily recruited, as are the *arms* and *hands*. In addition, the *quadriceps* are important in the deadlift, just as the glutes and hamstrings are important in the squat. The core must be rock-solid to allow the forces to be moved through the body. The core is more than just the abs—think of it as a cylinder circling the body that starts at the diaphragm and extends about halfway down the thighs. If that cylinder isn't kept tight, you'll never lift heavy. If the abs aren't braced, the risk of a back injury increases.

Push-ups

Push-ups are a horizontal pushing movement and probably the best-known and widely performed exercise ever. Depending on the placement of the hands, you'll work your chest or triceps. Push-ups work the *pectoralis major* and *minor* of the chest, the *deltoids* and the *triceps*, but doing push-ups properly requires full-body tension. If any body part isn't tight, the push-up will sag. Most people fail to activate the *gluteus maximus*, *hamstrings* and *abs* when doing push-ups, and you'll see their hips, waist or abs sagging and getting to the floor before the chest.

Box Jumps

Box jumps are an interesting movement. They're a partial squat with an explosive drive to hip extension on the way up. These, too, are a whole-body movement and many of my clients are amazed that their abs are sore the next day. Box jumps utilize the concept of stretch shortening. When you squat quickly, the *hamstrings* and *glutes* act like a spring: they compress and store energy, then they use that stored energy to drive you up explosively. This happens very fast in well under a second. You can test this for yourself. Start in a standing position; squat and hold at the bottom for 3 seconds, then jump as high as you can. Now do the same movement but don't pause at the bottom and see how much higher you can jump.

Jumping also uses the *quadriceps* and the muscles of the calves (the *soleus* and *gastrocnemius*), which generate power to spring up off the ground as well as absorb energy upon landing. The *abdominals* and the *hip flexors* are heavily recruited as the knees are brought up during the upward portion of the jump.

Floor Wipers

Floor wipers are a unique exercise that involves lying flat on your back while holding a barbell locked out. At the same time, the core has to be tight but also active as it brings the feet up from the floor to touch the plates on one side of the bar, lower them without touching the floor, then bring them up to the other side of the bar. So you have a static hold of the bar, active control of the core, including the quads, while at the same time allowing a bit of rotation to occur through the waist.

Because the floor wiper is actually several different exercises in one, it requires all the muscles of the body to work in unison. The static hold involves primarily the *pectoralis major* and *minor*, *triceps, anterior deltoids, latissimus dorsi* and *abdominals* (for stability). Many of the smaller back muscles are also involved in stabilizing the bar and torso. The leg movement uses the *hip flexors* (quadriceps and iliopsoas), the *rectus abdominis* and the *internal* and *external obliques*. The *hamstrings* and *gluteus maximus* are also utilized but in a more passive role of stabilization and control.

Dead Clean and Press

Kettlebell dead clean and press is two movements. The dead ("dead" meaning dead weight being lifted from the floor) clean (it "cleans" the body, never touching until coming to rest in the rack position) is a full-body exercise. It's primarily a squat type of movement, but also very explosive. Doing it right requires a lot of coordination from the ground up, but you also have to learn to be soft to minimize the impact of the bell on the back of the arm as it comes to the rack position, resting in the V of the arm with the elbow in the ribs. The dead clean is mostly about using the *quadriceps* and keeping the *core* solid; the *gluteus maximus* may come into play a bit. The shoulders, arms and hands are minimally involved. If you go heavy or do a lot of dead cleans, you'll feel it in your quads very quickly but you shouldn't feel it in your traps, upper back or arms, at least not until the next day.

The press portion of the dead clean and press is also a full-body movement. Contrary to what most gym rats will tell you, the press is not about how fast you can get the weight overhead. While the deltoids are recruited, they aren't the primary focus. The primary muscles involved are the *latissimus dorsi*, the *deltoids* and the *triceps*. In addition, you should also feel presses in the muscles that make up the *rotator cuff*, the *upper pectorals* and the *rhomboids*, plus your *abdominals, gluteus maximus* and *quadriceps*. Remember: The tighter you are throughout the entire body, the stronger you are (the principle of hyper-irradiation).

EQUIPMENT

To get the most out of the training programs in this book, you'll need to acquire or have access to a variety of tools for your exercise toolbox. Beyond the basics of a barbell, dumbbells and kettlebells, you'll need a pull-up bar, a sledgehammer, a heavy tire, a thick sandbag and heavy-duty resistance bands (not the flimsy tubing they sell at Target or Wal-Mart).

Barbell For the deadlift, you'll need a barbell. Olympic style is preferred, but if all you have is access to the standard size, that's ok. The Olympic barbell uses a bar that's thicker in diameter and taller plates. When using 45-pound plates, the bar is 9 inches off the floor. Standard plates are shorter, which makes the deadlift harder because you have to pull through a greater range of motion.

Kettlebell Kettlebells are a superior form of strength and endurance training. They're the perfect tool to teach the user how to utilize the entire body as a unit, making the whole body produce and apply force. These versatile pieces of equipment have been around since the 1700s, where they were purportedly used in Russia as a counterweight to measure grain. Somewhere along the way someone figured out they could be used for exercise, and they've been used for squats, presses, deadlifts, snatches, push-ups, pull-ups and countless other movements ever since.

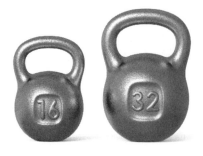

Because of their origin, kettlebells are weighted in kilograms; however, some American companies use pounds as the unit of measure. Throughout this book we'll use kilos as our unit of measure and give pounds in parentheses. Traditional weights are 8k (18 lb.), 12k (26 lb.), 16k (35 lb.), 24k (53 lb.), 32k (70 lb.) and 40k (88 lb.). Some companies have introduced bells to fill in the gaps between the traditional sizes so now you can also get bells in 10k (22 lb.), 14k (31 lb.), 20k (44 lb.), 28k (62 lb.) and 36k (79 lb.). At the very least you'll need a 16k bell for guys (as prescribed by the Spartan Warrior Workout for men) and an 8k for women. Stronger women may want to use 10 or 12k bells. If possible, try to get a second bell one size heavier.

Note that, unlike the dumbbell, the kettlebell is an offset weight. This offset center of mass makes many movements much more difficult and requires a lot more stabilization in certain positions. Many exercises are much more suited to kettlebells than dumbbells, such as the swing and the clean and snatch.

Dumbbell   Dumbbells are fairly easy to come by. All gyms have them and they're available at any sporting goods or department store. You'll need to have several, and in pairs, if possible. The weights you'll need depend on your strength levels; women may want to start at 5 pounds, men may start at 20 pounds. You may elect to go up in either 5- or 10-pound increments.

Lifting Chalk   Lifting chalk improves your grip in pull-ups, deadlifts and the dead clean and press by increasing friction in your hand. It's magnesium—NOT the same chalk used for playing pool—and is available at sporting-goods and outdoor/climbing stores.

Sandbag   The sandbag, used for the clean and press, can be made easily with a duffle bag or other heavy canvas bag, playground sand and some heavy-duty plastic contractor's bags. You can also buy them online.

Clothing & Shoes   Using a running shoe or a cross-trainer will not give you the support you need when doing the deadlifts and clean and presses. Normally we prefer to train barefoot whenever possible, but because you'll be doing box jumps, you should wear shoes to protect your feet from getting banged when landing on the box. We recommend Army or other flat, sturdy boots or old-school high- or low-top basketball shoes (aka "Chucks").

Your pants or shorts should be loose enough to move in but not baggy; the extra material will get in the way of certain movements. Tops (T-shirts, tank tops) should be comfortable—not baggy or super tight. Wearing clothing made of "wick away" material will help keep you cool and dry, especially in warmer months. Terrycloth sweat bands for your wrists not only help keep sweat from running down your arms onto your hand, making it tough to maintain your grip, they also reduce the pressure a kettlebell can place on the forearm when pressing and they provide padding while learning the dead clean movement, which can bang you up until you get the technique down.

TRAINING JOURNAL

In order to track your progress throughout the course of the Spartan Warrior Workout, you should log each workout, noting the weights used, number of reps/sets performed and how you felt before, during and after each workout. The journal will let you see how far you've come.

Spartan Nutrition

In order to train like a Spartan, you'll need to apply the same dedication and discipline to your eating habits. Instead of thinking about how you eat as a "diet," try to change your mindset and look at it as modifying the way you eat to help you get the best fuel for your body. Thinking about food this way tends to make proper eating a lifetime habit rather than a six-week plan that you can come off of any time you don't feel like sticking with it. To get the most benefit from the Spartan Warrior Workout, you'll need to fuel the engine that is your body with healthy, nutritious food that isn't full of chemical preservatives, hormones or antibiotics.

WHAT TO EAT

Splitting your total caloric requirements across five or six meals per day will keep your insulin and energy levels steady—no more crashing after lunch because you ate too many carbs or just ate too much in general. You

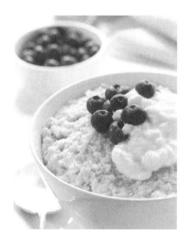

should eat approximately the same number of grams of carbs, proteins and fats at each meal. To get the most from your food dollars, try to buy and prepare your foods as *fresh* as possible (buy locally grown meats, vegetables and fruit when available and eat them soon), as *whole* as possible (cutting food causes them to start breaking down more quickly, causing nutrient degradation) and as *raw* as possible (in most cases, especially for vegetables, less cooked means more nutrients).

A good **breakfast** will give your body and brain the fuel it needs to get off to a good start. A high-quality carbohydrate like steel-cut oats provides your brain with energy; mix in some nuts for extra protein and berries for vitamins, antioxidants and fiber. An omelet with spinach or other veggies offers protein, good carbs and fiber; fruit on the side boosts your vitamin count. **Lunch** is typically when many people pig out, but a mid-morning snack should prevent you from doing so. For both lunch and **dinner**, try lean meat (chicken, beef, bison, turkey, fish), green veggies (spinach, broccoli, green beans), a little fruit and maybe some Greek yogurt.

Mid-morning and mid-afternoon snacks will prevent you from feeling like you're starving and will help you maintain an even energy level. A light protein, some nuts, an apple and yogurt work here. Depending on what time you had dinner, it's ok to have an **evening snack** an hour or so before bedtime. A low-carb snack of nuts and yogurt or cottage cheese is great.

You should strive to eat this way the majority of the time, even well after you've completed the Spartan Warrior Workout. However, there will be times when you're going to have that pizza, beer and ice cream. Cheat meals are okay as long as they only happen once a week. As with cheat meals, having a beer or a glass of wine occasionally while eating at a nice restaurant is ok, but know that alcohol will totally ruin your chances for a truly ripped body. So drink wisely and try to eliminate alcohol from your diet as much as possible.

Water, on the other hand, is something your body can't get enough of. Every part of your body—muscles, skin, kidneys, liver, brain, bones—requires water. Proper hydration reduces the chance of injuries and feelings of fatigue. Drink up to 64 ounces of water, although you may need more if you sweat a lot. You don't need anything fancy, like vitamin water. Drink filtered tap water or bottled spring water, but don't spend a fortune on it. A high-quality fish oil or krill oil should also be taken every day to minimize inflammation. It's also good for the joints, among other things.

Pre-/Post-Workout Recovery

When you're training hard, you can change up some of your meals for a pre-/post-workout recovery drink taken no more than an hour after your workout. This doesn't really count as a meal. The sugar and high carbs in a pre-/post-workout drink cause your insulin levels to spike (normally this is a problem as some of the sugar gets converted to fat and some gets burned off quickly, causing you to crash), but since your metabolism is increased post-exercise, the sugar is sucked into the energy systems, pulling the proteins with it and thus feeding the muscles what they need to get stronger and recover more quickly.

Recent studies have shown that low-fat chocolate milk is as good as, if not better than, any powder or "ready-to-drink" shake you can buy. The macronutrient ratio is ideal for replenishing the body after a hard workout. However, this doesn't mean you should drink a gallon of chocolate milk whenever you feel like. One or two 8-ounce glasses of low-fat chocolate milk is all you need, even better if it's organic milk. If you're lactose intolerant, stick with the powders. Look for one that's organic or natural and uses real sugar—not artificial sweetener or high fructose corn syrup. It may have some vitamins and minerals added to aid in recovery as well.

WHAT NOT TO EAT

Processed Foods   Processed foods such as most lunchmeats, pre-cooked meats, frozen dinners, chips, cookies and most other foods in the grocery store are processed. This just means that they have a bunch of junk added to them to keep them fresh longer or make them look and taste better. In most cases the food, which was full of nutrients, is stripped down to nothing, then things are added back in to make it "better." A good example is bread. All the fiber and nutrients are stripped from the wheat or rye when it's made into flour, then the vitamins and minerals that were naturally present get added back in, but now they're man-made, not natural.

If you read the label and see lots of ingredients that you can't pronounce, in most cases those are additives and preservatives and should be avoided.

Genetically Modified Foods   While the FDA and big farm conglomerates say GMO foods are safe, we really don't know. They haven't been around long enough to see conclusive results. Europe has extremely strict standards against GMOs, and in many countries they are banned.

I advise against eating non-organic beef, chicken, milk and other animal proteins. Hormone shots, antibiotics and other substances are given to these animals so the farms can get more meat out of fewer animals for less cost. However, we still don't know the full effects of what these "enhancers" do to humans. The FDA says they're safe, but other researchers contend that the rise in the use of hormones and antibiotics in animals seems to correspond to the increase in odd diseases like chronic fatigue syndrome, irritable bowel syndrome, fibromyalgia and a host of other diseases, which were unheard of even 60 years ago. I also recommend avoiding soy because in addition to the high levels of estrogen it contains, almost all soy is genetically modified.

Meal Replacement Drinks   If you're busy, you may not have time to fix every meal and snack. A meal replacement drink is a great option, but you need to read the labels—many MRDs have lots of junk and tons of sugar or artificial sweeteners, both of which you need to avoid. A good MRD should have 10–15 grams of fiber to help you feel full, some good carbs and a high-quality protein.

VITAMINS AND MINERALS

The main reason to take a quality multivitamin and mineral daily is that current farming methods have stripped a lot of nutrients from the soil so the foods we grow don't get them from the ground, and then we don't get them either.

The various brand-name multivitamin pills are mostly worthless. A good multivitamin should be liquid and needs to be refrigerated. Your body will absorb the liquid much more readily than a pill. Taking a liquid vitamin also allows you to adjust the dosage. It's ok to take a small dose twice a day to make sure you're getting enough of the vitamins while minimizing the amount of the vitamins your body is excreting.

MRDs are a quick fix, but use them only when there's no time. Even though they'll tide you over until the next meal, they're not a substitute for real food.

Sports Drinks   Drinks like Gatorade are just sugar water with some minerals added, and unless you're training intensely for hours at a time in the summer heat and humidity, all you need is water. The amount of sugar in Gatorade is massive. A 32-ounce bottle contains 14 grams (½ ounce) of sugar *per serving*. There are four servings per bottle for a whopping 56 grams (2 ounces) of sugar. Most people buy the 32-ounce bottle and suck it all down before they realize it (if they realize it at all). Your body cannot process that much sugar at once so it gets stored as fat. Even the G2 "low" carb version has 5 grams of sugar per serving, or 20 grams per bottle, which is still a lot.

The only other ingredients in Gatorade are water, sodium and potassium. Most people get plenty of sodium in their diet and don't train hard enough to add more. Instead of potassium what you probably need is a good magnesium powder if you cramp a lot in your feet or calves. Magnesium deficiency can cause all sorts of problems, from angina to constipation, headaches and migraines, insulin resistance, PMS, leg cramps, muscle twitches and more. Magnesium also helps the body use calcium. Without magnesium, the build-up of calcium in the blood manifests as arrhythmia, angina, hypertension and migraines.

MAINTAINING A HEALTHY DIET

Most people follow a program of diet and exercise for six weeks or six months then "fall off the wagon" and gain back all the fat they lost and wind up being in worse shape than ever. Don't let that happen to you. You'll work your ass off doing the training programs in this book. Don't lose your hard-earned progress by reverting to your past ways.

Adhering to the following guidelines throughout the course of your Spartan training will help you get stronger and build your stamina tremendously—and as a byproduct you'll get ripped. But don't go back to your old eating habits after you've conquered the Spartan Warrior Workout. Keep eating this same way and you'll feel better and be better able to maintain your Spartan physique over time.

Do...

Eat breakfast every morning. Have some good carbs like steel-cut oatmeal (not that instant junk with all the additives and sugars) or muesli, or eat an omelet with a little lean meat and veggies.

Eat lots of fresh vegetables. Try to have some at every meal, especially the green ones. Remember that white potatoes aren't veggies, and neither is corn (it's a grain).

Eat a lot of fresh fruit. Apples, dates, oranges and bananas are all good options.

Eat good proteins. Have lean meat, like turkey, chicken and fish, or nuts, like almonds and cashews.

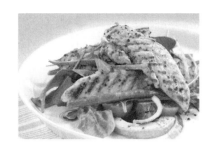

Drink a gallon of water per day. You may need more if you sweat a lot.

Take a high-quality fish oil. Liquid is preferable; keep it refrigerated.

Take a high-quality liquid multivitamin and mineral. This will help ensure your body gets everything it needs.

Eat organic food when possible. It's even better if it's locally grown, too.

Don't...

Eat any "white" food. No breads, white potatoes, pasta or rice.

Eat artificial foods or sweeteners. If you need sweetener in your coffee, try raw sugar, agave nectar or stevia. Instead of artificial creamer, use real cream or half-and-half.

Eat fast food. No McDonald's or Wendy's. No Taco Bell, Quiznos or Subway either. Read the fine print at the bottom of their ads (assuming you can read print that small) and you'll see that the results of the people who lost weight eating those foods were not normal. The Taco Bell "Diet" is the biggest hoax going.

Eat processed foods. They're loaded with salt and preservatives. This includes TV dinners, even Weight Watchers and Lean Cuisine meals.

In General, Remember...

Eat five to six small meals per day. Make sure you get some protein, veggies and fruit at each meal.

Don't take supplements (other than fish oil, multivitamins and minerals). They're meant to add to the nutrition you get from real food, not to replace it.

Active Rest and Cycling Your Training

In order for your body to continue tackling challenges such as the Spartan Warrior Workout, you'll need to give it some TLC—or better yet, active rest/recovery. Active rest or active recovery means taking a day off but still being active. Basically, you do something very light and different from your regular workouts. It could be something as simple as a nice stroll (*not* a brisk walk) through the park, light gardening, easy biking (if your main exercise doesn't include biking), tai chi or other gentle movements, including light yoga. By staying active on an off day, you keep fresh blood pumping to the muscles, lubricate the joints and help to reduce soreness and stiffness. The worst thing you can do when taking a day off is to sit around in front of the TV, especially after a really hard workout, regardless of whether it was a heavy strength day or a day of high-intensity interval training (HIIT).

Active rest helps your body to reset itself and, if folded into your training regime, it will allow you to train better and harder the next time you hit the gym. Your training is cyclical in nature, just like everything else. Our bodies have days when everything is working 100 percent, and other days when we may feel like we're only functioning at 75 percent. By taking this cycle into account, we can try to sync our training with our natural rhythms and take advantage of them.

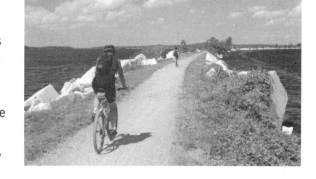

One method you can try is moving from a moderate day to a strength day, followed by a high-intensity day and then an active-recovery no-intensity day. During this cycle you should focus on making improvements in one area, such as improving your pull-ups; everything in your workouts would revolve around this specific goal. This cycle can be followed forever if you want to since it has everything you need to stay healthy and injury free.

Other cycles tend to follow a bodybuilder routine: train three or four times per week (such as Monday, Tuesday, off Wednesday, then train on Thursday and Friday), doing body part splits like chest and back one day, biceps and triceps another day. On the off days, the trainee may do nothing or light to moderate cardio, such as the elliptical.

Regardless of the training cycle you choose, you should always go by how you feel. If you're having a tough day and the weight feels heavy, back off a little and don't do as many reps; if it's a HIIT day, slow down a little and don't push quite as hard. On those days when you feel ready to take on the world, go for it. Kick some ass.

With the Spartan Warrior Workout, because we're trying to train six different exercises at the same time, we have to take a slightly different approach: trying to work similar movements on the same day (once you've hit the intermediate level) and keeping exercises that support the other lifts but at a low to moderate intensity. There are some active recovery days built into the schedule, so be sure to use them appropriately. Don't try to skip a planned recovery day—you'll only wind up losing ground or, worse, getting injured.

During the course of following the programs in this book, remember to listen to your body. If you aren't up to the intensity of that day's workout, back off a little—but not too much though. No slackers allowed. To get the results you want, you have to train hard, but you also have to be smart as well. We don't want you to sustain any injuries or aggravate any you may have incurred in the past.

PART 2

The Programs

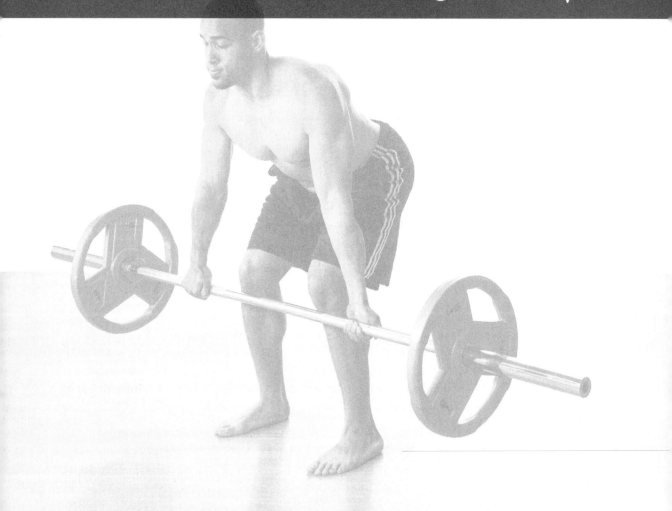

Programs Overview

This section lays out in exact detail the two programs that will take you from a rank beginner in the Spartan Warrior Workout to top performer. Prepare yourself, though: This training is not for the weak of body or mind. It'll be very tough and will require you to train even when you feel like crap. Place your mind inside the warrior of the era—if you give up, whine, quit or don't give 100 percent, you die!

Program 1 is for people with little to no experience in the weight room. You'll need to learn the movements and be able to do them correctly before you start going full blast. This program uses many assistance exercises that will help you perfect your technique in the six Spartan Warrior Workout exercises.

For this program, you'll train four days per week, whether it's Monday through Thursday, Monday/Wednesday/Friday/Sunday, or some other combination of days. Just make sure to rest three days out of the week. This program will push you hard and you'll quickly see improvements across the board. However, don't neglect joint mobility and stretching (see pages 123–46) to maintain/improve flexibility and minimize risk of injury; this should be done on your off-days as well.

ACRONYMS

The following are a few key acronyms you'll come across in the programs:

ALAP - as long as possible

AMRAP - as many reps as possible

AQAP - as quickly as possible

DB - dumbbell

KB - kettlebell

1RM - 1 rep max

Program 2 is for people who've been training with free weights and body weight for at least six months and have a decent level of overall fitness. In order to compress this 28-day training cycle, rest periods are built in. So unlike Program 1, you should train every day if you can. During the course of this cycle, you'll have two occasions (days 14 and 29) to do the actual Spartan Warrior Workout. To ensure that you'll be fresh for your attempt and then give you a day to recover before continuing your training, we've programmed in an "active rest" day before and after both of these test days.

Occasionally you'll come across a section that looks like this:

	LEVEL	MOVEMENT	SETS	REPS/TIME/INTERVAL	REST	COMMENTS
1	All	Pull-Ups *p. 47*		25		AQAP; do in chunks
2	All	Deadlifts *p. 55*	10	5	1 min	85% of 1RM
3	1	*Incline Push-Ups *p. 67*	2	10	20 sec	
	2	*Decline Push-Ups *p. 77*	2	10	20 sec	
	3	*Decline Push-Ups *p. 77*	2	10	20 sec	if easy, add weight vest
4	All	*Low Windmills *p. 108*	2	8 each side	30 sec	men 24k, women 16k
5	All	*RFESS *p. 84*	3	10 each side	30 sec	2 KB/DB hanging down; men 16k, women 12k
6	All	*Sandbag Clean & Press *p. 97*	3	8	1 min	heavy weight: minimum 50lb men (70 preferably), 25lb women (35 preferably)
	Optional Circuit: Do starred exercises for 30 sec each (30 sec each side where applicable, no rest between sides, *but* alternate sides with Sandbag Clean & Press); 30 sec rest between exercises; 4 rounds total					
7	All	Inverted or Ring Rows *p. 52*	5	10	1 min	use weight vest if you're strong enough
		Sled Push *p. 115*	2	100 ft	1 min	go heavy

Here you have the option to do a portion of the workout as a high-intensity interval training (HIIT) circuit. Don't do both ways. Doing a circuit is much tougher than performing the exercises on a sets/reps basis. It minimizes your rest, which will improve your endurance and strengthen your cardiovascular system. On days you feel sluggish, skip the circuit.

If you don't choose to do the circuit, do the workout one exercise at a time, following the prescribed sets/reps/ rest: 2 sets of 10 push-ups at the appropriate level with 20 seconds of rest between sets, followed by 2 sets of 8 low windmills (do 8 on each side before taking a 30-second rest), 3 sets of 10 RFESS (do 10 on each side before taking a 30-second rest), and finally 3 sets of 8 sandbag cleans and presses with 1 minute of rest between sets.

If you do choose to do the circuit, you'd do push-ups for 30 seconds, rest for 30 seconds, do low windmills, rest for 30 seconds, do RFESS (30 seconds per side), rest for 30 seconds, and finally do the sandbag clean and press (alternating sides each rep) for 30 seconds. You'd perform this circuit 4 times.

By the time you complete Level 2, you should be able to conquer the workout. We want you to be able to do the Spartan Warrior Workout quickly (20 minutes or less), but we also want to keep you safe and healthy. Don't try to beat the clock by training with sloppy technique; you *will* get injured. Take your time and perfect the exercises. Remember: It's about the quality of movement, not the quantity or the speed.

A FEW TRAINING NOTES

Before you start either program, first make sure you've determined your 1 RMs (see page 56 for the deadlift and page 90 for the bench press). You'll need those numbers to calculate your working load (e.g., 50% of 1 RM). You'll also want to figure out your pull-up and push-up levels: *beginners* can do 0–5 push/pull-ups, *intermediates* 5–15, *advanced* 15+.

Next, make sure you warm up before each workout, doing joint mobility drills and a light bodyweight circuit as described on page 122. Just a brisk, 2- to 3-minute non-stop routine will suffice.

Specified weights are a recommended minimum, especially when it's stated as a heavy lift. For "light weight," use a weight one size less than your usual kettlebell or 10 pounds less than your dumbbell (for example, women who press 8k should use either a 6k kettlebell or 12-lb. dumbbell, men who press 16k should use a 12k kettlebell or 26-lb. dumbbell); for "heavy weight," go up at least one size from your usual, especially for lower body work.

The "finisher" is extra work, sometimes to amplify your workload in a specific exercise, but typically to increase your endurance and mental toughness. If you feel you're not getting enough work on certain exercises (such as pull-ups), you can do the workout for that exercise again.

Training Concepts

These programs use several training protocols alongside traditional sets and reps: ladders, density training, negatives and tempo lifts. Each method evokes a different response from the body; cycling through a variety of stimuli keeps you from getting bored and your body from plateauing.

Ladders can be ascending and descending. With an *ascending ladder,* you perform an exercise for a certain number of reps; this is a rung on the ladder. For the next set/rung, you add 1 rep (or 2, in some cases); on the third set/rung, you add yet another rep. The reps scheme looks like this: 1/2/3/4/5/6/7/8/9/10. This is 55 total reps (or 55 reps per side for unilateral exercises). Ascending ladders build endurance; you may start with a moderately heavy weight and stick with it on all rungs, but you'll probably find that you have to drop the weight as you climb the ladder.

The *descending ladder* is the exact opposite: Start at the top of the ladder and go down to the bottom one rung at a time, or 10/9/8/7/6/5/4/3/2/1 (55 reps per side if you complete the entire ladder). Descending ladders build strength; as you go down, you should increase the poundage until you're performing close to a 1 RM lift on the last rung.

When ascending the ladder, you should take a slightly longer rest as you climb up. During a descending ladder, the rest should decrease each rung.

Density training tries to pack a lot of work into a short time frame with a workload that you can handle each interval. Density training works well for increasing your rep count in high-rep exercises like pull-ups and push-ups; however, you need to be able to consistently do at least 3 to 5 reps of whichever exercise(s) you're trying to improve.

Let's set a goal of 25 pull-ups since it's the number required in the Spartan Warrior Workout. The protocol requires us to double this number to 50. To determine the reps and intervals, take the number of good pull-ups you can do in one set when fresh, then subtract 2 from that to get a starting point. Let's assume you can get 5 good pull-ups in one set; by subtracting 2, we get 3 reps for a starting point. If you can do 10, start the training at the 8-rep mark.

Here's a sample table to see how density training works.

Total Reps: 50; starting reps: 3

- 3 reps every minute on the minute for 20 minutes
- 4 reps every minute on the minute for 12 minutes
- 5 reps every minute on the minute for 10 minutes
- 6 reps every minute on the minute for 9 minutes
- 7 reps every minute on the minute for 8 minutes
- 8 reps every minute on the minute for 7 minutes
- 9 reps every minute on the minute for 6 minutes
- 10 reps every minute on the minute for 5 minutes
- 11 reps every minute on the minute for 5 minutes
- 12 reps every minute on the minute for 4 minutes
- 15 reps every minute on the minute for 4 minutes
- 16 reps every minute on the minute for 3 minutes
- 18 reps every minute on the minute for 3 minutes
- 20 reps every minute on the minute for 2 minutes

At this point you should be able to knock out 25 pull-ups in one set. Of course, this isn't going to happen over-night; it can take months or even a year to get to this stage. The secret is hard work and not to rush things. If you move from 10 pull-ups to 11 pull-ups and fail at any point in the 11-rep-per-minute set, you should not go to 12 until you can get 11 easily and consistently.

Density training is very tough on the nervous system so don't use it more than twice per week for the same exercise, but you can use it for two or more exercises at the same time, say, pull-ups in one 20-minute block and push-ups in another, twice per week.

Another example would be the 50 push-up mark. We'll assume you can do 15 good reps; subtract 2 and you'll start with 13.

- 13 reps every minute on the minute for 8 minutes
- 15 reps every minute on the minute for 7 minutes
- 20 reps every minute on the minute for 5 minutes
- 25 reps every minute on the minute for 4 minutes
- 30 reps every minute on the minute for 3 minutes +10 (to get to 100)
- 40 reps every minute on the minute for 2 minutes +20 (to get to 100)

At this point doing 50 at once should be no problem.

Negatives (or eccentrics) will build your strength quickly. The slow lowering of a very heavy weight (or your body weight) causes muscles to contract much harder than when picking up the weight or pulling/pushing yourself. Your body responds to these contractions by making the muscle fibers stronger and bigger to better handle the overload. Due to the intense focus involved in doing negatives, it's best to only do a few at a time until your body and your central nervous system get used to them.

For negative pull-ups, get your chin over the bar any way you can (by jumping or getting a boost) then slowly lower down to a dead hang. Your strength will diminish rapidly, but you'll get stronger quickly and be able to do more full reps even if you can't do one pull-up. For negative push-ups (regardless of starting position), slowly lower yourself with good form until your chest is almost on the floor, then go to your knees, return to the top position and repeat. As you get stronger, go more slowly or add a weight vest to make it more difficult.

Tempo lifts increase your time under tension (TUT)—the longer your body remains under tension during an exercise, the stronger it will become. In these programs you might see push-ups written as "5-count lower/raise/rest" or pull-ups noted as "1-count up/down, 3-count hold at top." The first has you take 5 seconds to lower down toward the floor, hold at the bottom for 5 seconds and take 5 seconds to come back up. The second has you take one second to pull up, hold your chin above the bar for 3 seconds and take one second to lower down.

LEVEL		MOVEMENT	SETS	REPS/TIME/INTERVAL	REST	COMMENTS
1	1	Dead Hang *p. 49*	2	ALAP	1 min	
		Supported Pull-Up *p. 50*	3	5	1 min	
	2	Density Pull-Up *p. 47*	20	3 every min on the min		
	3	Pull-Up *p. 47*		5/4/3/2/1	breaths = # reps done	
		Inverted Row *p. 52*	5	10	30 sec	
2	All	Deadlift *p. 55*	5	5	1 min	use empty bar or 50% of 1RM
3	1	Static Hold (Top) *p. 69*	5	ALAP	30 sec	
		Static Hold (Bottom) *p. 69*	5	ALAP	30 sec	try to do this every hour throughout the day
	2	Push-Up *p. 67*	5	AMRAP	1 min	
		Static Hold (Bottom) *p. 69*	5	1 min	30 sec	
		Static Hold (Middle) *p. 69*	5	1 min	30 sec	
	3	Push-Up *p. 67*	1	AMRAP		
4	All	Static Lunge *p. 83*	5	20 sec/leg	20 sec *after* 2nd leg	
5	All	High Plank *p. 93*	5	30 sec	30 sec	
6	All	Dead Clean & Press *p. 97*	3	10 each arm	30 sec	moderate weight
7	All	Sledgehammer *p. 113*	1	50		stand in a square stance
		Squat Thrust *p. 136*	8	20 sec	10 sec	rest in high plank

LEVEL		MOVEMENT	SETS	REPS/TIME/INTERVAL	REST	COMMENTS
1	All	Dead Hang *p. 49*	2	ALAP	30 sec	
		Inverted Row *p. 52*	3	5	30 sec	
		Half Pull-Up (lower half) *p. 51*	1	AMRAP		
		Static Hold: Chin over Bar *p. 49*	1	ALAP		
2	All	Deadlift *p. 55*	5	10	1 min	60% of 1RM
		2-Hand KB Swing *p. 59*	5	30 sec	30 sec	heavy weight
		Hip Extension *p. 61*	3	10	30 sec	pause at top
3	1	Chest Touch *p. 74*	8	20 sec work/ 10 sec rest	1 min *after* finishing entire circuit	
		Static Hold (Bottom) *p. 69*	5	ALAP	minimal	
	2	KB Floor Press *p. 75*	5	10	30 sec	2 bells
		Renegade Row *p. 74*	5	10	30 sec	2 bells
	3	Up Dog into Down Dog *p. 141*	5	30 sec	30 sec	
4	All	Jump Squat *p. 81*	8	20 sec work/ 10 sec rest		keep toes on floor
5	All	Bench Press *p. 89*	2	10	30 sec	light weight; intermediate push-up level can skip this
6	All	Dead Clean *p. 97*	3	10 each arm	30 sec	moderate weight
7	All	Ab Rollout *p. 121*	3	5		from knees
		Farmer's Walk *p. 118*	3	100 ft	1 min	go heavy, one bell in each hand

1 PULL-UP   **2** DEADLIFT   **3** PUSH-UP   **4** BOX JUMP   **5** FLOOR WIPER   **6** DEAD CLEAN & PRESS   **7** FINISHER

	LEVEL	MOVEMENT	SETS	REPS/TIME/INTERVAL	REST	COMMENTS
1	All	1-Arm Supported Row p. 76	6	30 sec/arm	30 sec *after* 2nd arm	
2	All	Deadlift p. 55	3	5	30 sec	50% of 1RM
3	1	*Circuit:* KB Floor Press p. 75/ Single KB Floor Press p. 75/ KB Floor Press: Static Hold p. 75	1	30 sec each item	2 min *after* completing circuit	
	2	Push-Up p. 67	1	AMRAP		
	3	Push-Up p. 67		10/9/8/7/6/5/4/3/2/1	1 min *after* completing ladder	
		High Plank p. 69	3	10	30 sec	
		Walkout p. 134	3	10	30 sec	
4	All	Goblet Squat p. 101	1	10		moderate weight
5	All	Unicycle p. 96	5	30 sec/side	30 sec *after* 2nd side	
		Floor Press: Static Hold p. 89	1		ALAP	light barbell or bells
6	All	Dead Clean & Press p. 97	5	30 sec/arm	30 sec	moderate weight
7	All	Tire Flip p. 112	5	5	1 min	heavy weight

	LEVEL	MOVEMENT	SETS	REPS/TIME/INTERVAL	REST	COMMENTS
1	1	Dead Hang p. 49	1	ALAP	30 sec	
		Half Pull-Up (lower half) p. 51	1	ALAP	30 sec	
	2	Density Pull-Up p. 47	20	3 every min on the min		If Day 1 was easy, do 15 sets of 4 in 15 min. If Day 1 was too hard, do 20 sets of 2 in 20 minutes.
	3	Inverted Row p. 52	8	20 sec	10 sec	
2	All	1-Leg Deadlift p. 62	6	30 sec/leg	30 sec *after* 2nd leg	
3	1	Push-Up p. 67	1	AMRAP		from knees if necessary
	2	Incline Push-Up p. 78	1	AMRAP		
	3	Push-Up p. 67	1	AMRAP		
4	All	Jump Tuck p. 82	8	20 sec	10 sec	
		Step-Up p. 85	5	30 sec alternating legs	30 sec	use same box height you are jumping to
5	All	KB Floor Press p. 91	3	5	30 sec	barbell or 2 moderate bells; 1-count up/down, 3-count hold at top
6	All	Press p. 97	5	3 each arm	30 sec	heavy weight
		Dead Clean p. 97	5	5 each arm	30 sec	heavy weight
7	1	Squat Thrust p. 136 or Burpee Level 1 p. 116	3	10	30 sec	
	2	Burpee Level 3 p. 117	3	10	30 sec	
	3	Burpee Level 5 p. 117	3	10	20 sec	

1 PULL-UP   2 DEADLIFT   3 PUSH-UP   4 BOX JUMP   5 FLOOR WIPER   6 DEAD CLEAN & PRESS   7 FINISHER

	LEVEL	MOVEMENT	SETS	REPS/TIME/INTERVAL	REST	COMMENTS
1	1	Static Hold: Chin over Bar p. 49	2	ALAP	30 sec	
	2	Static Hold: Chin over Bar p. 49	3	ALAP	30 sec	
	3	Static Hold: Chin over Bar p. 49	5	ALAP	20 sec	
2	All	1-Hand KB Swing p. 60	6	30 sec/arm	30 sec	
3	1	Partial Lower/Raise p. 70	1	AMRAP until form breaks	2 min	partial lower with 3-sec count; partial raise with 3-sec count after rest
	2	Push-Up p. 67	1	1 more than last time		
		Static Hold (Bottom) p. 69	5	1 min	30 sec	
	3	Mountain Climbers p. 114	5	30 sec	30	
4	All	Bodyweight Squat p. 100	8	20	10	
5	All	Floor Wiper p. 87	5	10	30 sec	use same weight as yesterday
		Unicycle p. 96	3	30 sec/side	30 sec	
		Static Hold p. 89	3	ALAP	1 min	
6	All	H2H Sumo Squat p. 103	5	30	30 sec	move quickly
7	1	Sled Push p. 115	3	50 ft	as needed	go heavy

	LEVEL	MOVEMENT	SETS	REPS/TIME/INTERVAL	REST	COMMENTS
1	All	Negative Pull-Up p. 47	3	AMRAP	30 sec	go down slowly
2	All	Suitcase Deadlift p. 63	5	30	30	2 bells
3	1	Incline Push-Up p. 78		AMRAP (not to failure)	1 min	
	2	Push-Up p. 67		AMRAP then −1	5 sec	descending ladder
	3	5-Count Push-Up p. 67	1	10		5-count lower/raise/rest
4	All	RFESS p. 84	5	20 sec	20 sec after 2nd leg	
5	All	Leg Thrust p. 92	3	10	30 sec	
6	All	Dead Clean & Press p. 97	5	20 sec/arm	20 sec after 2nd arm	use 70% 1RM or 1 size down
7	All	Sandbag Shoulder p. 99	5	10	1 min	heavy weight; alternate sides each rep

	LEVEL	MOVEMENT	SETS	REPS/TIME/INTERVAL	REST	COMMENTS
1	1	Supported Pull-Up p. 50	3	AMRAP	30 sec	
		Dead Hang p. 49	3	ALAP	30 sec	
	2 & 3	Density Pull-Up p. 47	20	3 every min on the min		If Day 4 was easy, do 10 sets of 5 in 10 min. Otherwise do this.
2	All	Deadlift p. 55	5	10	30 sec	barbell 50% of 1RM
3	1	Renegade Row p. 74	8	20	10	switch sides during rest
	2 & 3	Push-Up p. 67		AMRAP in 5 min	as needed	
4	All	Jump Squat p. 81	1	15	30 sec	
5	All	Bench Press p. 89	3	10	30 sec	50% of 1RM
		Leg Raise p. 92	3	10	30 sec	
6	All	Dead Clean & Press p. 97	1	10		moderate KB/DB
7	All	Band Row p. 119	5	30 sec	15 sec	

LEVEL		MOVEMENT	SETS	REPS/TIME/INTERVAL	REST	COMMENTS
1	All	Inverted Row *p. 52*	3	10	30 sec	
2	All	Deadlift *p. 55*	5	20	30 sec	barbell 50% of 1RM
		2-Hand KB Swing *p. 59*	5	10	30 sec	heavy weight
3	1 & 2	REST				
	3	High Plank *p. 69*	5	10	30 sec	
4	All	Goblet Squat *p. 101*	5	40	20 sec	moderate KB/DB
5	All	Static Hold *p. 89*	3	ALAP	1 min	barbell 90% of 1RM
6	All	Dead Clean *p. 97*	3	10 each side	30 sec	light to moderate KB/DB
		Press *p. 97*	3	10 each side	30 sec	light to moderate KB/DB
7	All	High Plank *p. 93*	5	ALAP	30 sec	
		Mountain Climbers *p. 114*	8	20	10 sec	

LEVEL		MOVEMENT	SETS	REPS/TIME/INTERVAL	REST	COMMENTS
1	1 & 2	1-Arm Supported Row *p. 53*	3	10 each side	30 sec	heavy KB/DB
	3	Jumping Pull-Up *p. 52*	1	10		
2	All	High Pull *p. 66*	10/12/14/16/18/20/10		see notes	Rest no more than the time it took to do both arms at that rung of the ladder (use a stopwatch). After 20 per arm, do 10 per arm for a total of 100 reps per arm.
3	1	Static Hold (Top) *p. 69*	1	ALAP	30 sec	
		Static Hold (Bottom) *p. 69*	1	ALAP	30 sec	
		Static Hold (Middle) *p. 69*	1	ALAP	1 min	
		Partial Raise from Low Plank *p. 70*	1	AMRAP	30 sec	
		Partial Lower from High Plank *p. 70*		descending ladder starting with AMRAP	minimal	AMRAP/AMRAP-1/AMRAP-2/etc. until you get to 1
	2	Push Up *p. 67*		ascending ladder	minimal	continue until you can't complete a rung
	3	Push-Up *p. 67*		AMRAP in 5 min	as needed	rest 3–5 min before doing next exercise
4	All	Bodyweight Squat *p. 100*	8	20 sec	10 sec	
5	All	Leg Thrust *p. 92*	1	20		
6	All	Barbell Overhead Static Hold *p. 121*	3	ALAP	1 min	moderate weight
7	All	Tire/Sled Pull *p. 115*	3	100 ft	1 min	use light tire/sled and sprint

1 PULL-UP　　**2** DEADLIFT　　**3** PUSH-UP　　**4** BOX JUMP　　**5** FLOOR WIPER　　**6** DEAD CLEAN & PRESS　　**7** FINISHER

	LEVEL	MOVEMENT	SETS	REPS/TIME/INTERVAL	REST	COMMENTS
1	1	Static Hold: Chin over Bar *p. 49*	5	ALAP	30 sec	
	2 & 3	Pull-Up *p. 47*	varies	varies		If you can do 15 sets of 5 in 15 min without struggling, do that; if you can't, drop down to 16 sets of 4 in 16 min
2	All	Sumo Deadlift *p. 65*	5	30 sec	30 sec	heavy weight
3	1	*Circuit:* KB Floor Press *p. 75/* Single KB Floor Press *p. 75/* KB Floor Press: Static Hold *p. 75*	1	30 sec each item	2 min *after* completing circuit	
		Static Hold (Bottom) *p. 69*	1	ALAP	2 min	
		Triangle Push-Up *p. 77*	1	AMRAP		
	2	KB Floor Press *p. 75*	5	10	30 sec	
		Renegade Row *p. 95*	5	10 alternating sides	1 min	
	3	Static Hold (Top) *p. 69*	5	ALAP	30 sec	
4	All	Box Jump *p. 79*	1	50	as needed	AQAP; as high a box as possible
5	All	Russian Twist *p. 96*	5	30 sec	30 sec	
6	All	Sandbag Clean to Press *p. 106*	2	10	45 sec	60% of max weight
7	All	Sledgehammer *p. 113*	1	50 alternating sides		

	LEVEL	MOVEMENT	SETS	REPS/TIME/INTERVAL	REST	COMMENTS
1	1	Supported Pull-Up *p. 50*	1	AMRAP		
	2	Pull-Up *p. 47*	1	AMRAP		
	3	Pull-Up *p. 47*	1	AMRAP		
2	All	2-Hand KB Swing *p. 59*	3	15	20 sec	
3	1	Renegade Row *p. 95*	5	5 alternating sides	1 min	2 KB/DB; rest 2 min before moving to next exercise
	2	10-Count Push-Up *p. 67*	2	AMRAP	1 min	10-count down/hold/up
	3	Push-Up *p. 67*	1	AMRAP		
4	All	Step-Up *p. 85*	3	10 each side	30 sec	don't alternate legs
5	All	Floor Wiper *p. 87*	3	15	45 sec	70% of 1RM, or 95 for guys, 65 gals
		Leg Raise *p. 92*	3	10	30 sec	
6	All	Windmill *p. 108*	3	10 each side	30 sec	
7	All	Sledgehammer *p. 113*	1	50 alternating sides		stand in square stance

	LEVEL	MOVEMENT	SETS	REPS/TIME/INTERVAL	REST	COMMENTS
1	1	Band Row *p. 119*	5	20	30 sec	use tough but doable resistance
	2	Inverted Row *p. 52*	5	10	30 sec	as close to parallel to the floor as possible
	3	Pull-Up *p. 47*	2	5	30 sec	commando grip; switch grips after 5
2	All	Deadlift *p. 55*		10/9/8/7/6/5/4/3/2/1		barbell; start with easy weight then increase weight while decreasing reps
3	1	Incline Push-Up *p. 78*	5	AMRAP but not to failure	1 min	as little incline as possible
		High Plank *p. 69*	5	ALAP	30 sec	
	2/3	Walking Push-Up *p. 71*	5	10	30 sec	
4	All	Jump Tuck *p. 82*	2	20	45 sec	
5	All	KB Floor Press *p. 91*	2	10	20 sec	2 moderate KB/DB
6	All	Dead Clean & Press *p. 97*	3	20	20 sec	2 KB; 16k for men, 8k for women
7	All	*Circuit:* Overhead Static Hold *p. 121*/Double KB Rack Walk *p. 118*/Farmer's Walk *p. 118*	3	30 sec each item	1 min *after* each set	

	LEVEL	MOVEMENT	SETS	REPS/TIME/INTERVAL	REST	COMMENTS
1	1	Supported Pull-Up *p. 50*	3	10	30 sec	try to minimize the use of legs
	2	Density Pull-Up *p. 47*	varies	varies		If you can do 15 sets of 5 in 15 min without struggling, do that; if you can't, drop down to 16 sets of 4 in 16 min
	3	Pull-Up *p. 47*	1	15	minimal rest when necessary	
2	All	*Circuit:* 2-Hand KB Swing *p. 59*/Right 1-Hand Swing/Left 1-Hand Swing *p. 60*/H2H KB Swing *p. 61*	5	30 sec of each swing	1 min *after* 2 min of work	
3	1	REST				
	2	Push-Up *p. 67*	1	AMRAP		
	3	Walking Push-Up *p. 71*	2	30 sec	30 sec	
4	All	Mountain Climbers *p. 114*	8	20 sec	10 sec	
5	All	Leg Thrust *p. 92*	1	AMRAP		
6	All	Windmill + Overhead Squat *p. 109*		1 min/side		light weight; at top of windmill, do a squat
7	All	Burpees Level 5 *p. 117*	8	20 sec	10 sec	

1 PULL-UP **2** DEADLIFT **3** PUSH-UP **4** BOX JUMP **5** FLOOR WIPER **6** DEAD CLEAN & PRESS **7** FINISHER

LEVEL		MOVEMENT	SETS	REPS/TIME/INTERVAL	REST	COMMENTS
1	1	1-Arm Supported Row *p. 53*	5	10 each side	30 sec	heavy KB/DB; rest 1 min before doing Inverted Rows
		Inverted Row *p. 52*	3	10	45 sec	
	2 & 3	Renegade Row *p. 74*	3	10 alternating arms	30 sec	KB/DB
2	All	Deadlift *p. 55*		25	as needed	75% of 1RM, or 135lb for men, 95lb for women
3	1	Push-Up *p. 67*	1	AMRAP		
	2 & 3	High Plank *p. 69*	1	ALAP		
4	All	RFESS *p. 84*	5	20 sec	20 sec *after* 2nd leg	2 KB/DB at 80% of 1RM
5	All	Static Hold *p. 89*	2	ALAP	1 min	80% of 1RM
6	All	Press *p. 97*	5	5 each side	1 min	KB; 80% of 1RM
		Dead Clean *p. 97*	5	5	1 min	2 KB; 80% of 1RM
7	All	Band Row *p. 119*	5	30	15	

LEVEL		MOVEMENT	SETS	REPS/TIME/INTERVAL	REST	COMMENTS
1	All	Band Row *p. 119*	8	20 sec	10 sec	
2	All	Suitcase Deadlift *p. 63*	2	10	30 sec	2 light to moderate KB
3	1	Incline Push-Up *p. 78*	3	10	1 min	as little incline as possible
	2 & 3	Push-Up *p. 67*	1	25	minimal	
4	All	Bodyweight Squat *p. 100*	2	30 sec	30 sec	
5	All	Russian Twist *p. 96*	5	30 sec	30 sec	with KB/DB
6	All	Overhead Squat *p. 105*	3	8 each side	30 sec	70% of 1RM
7	All	Sledgehammer *p. 113*	5	30 sec alternating sides	30 sec	stand in a square stance

LEVEL		MOVEMENT	SETS	REPS/TIME/INTERVAL	REST	COMMENTS
1	All	Negative Pull-Up *p. 47*	1	AMRAP		
2	All	2-Hand KB Swing *p. 59*	1	20		light weight
3	1	Push-Up *p. 67*	1	AMRAP		
	2 & 3	Triangle Push-Up *p. 77*	1	AMRAP		
4	All	Box Jump *p. 79*	1	25		as tall a box as possible
5	All	Leg Raise *p. 92*	1	10		
6	All	Dead Clean *p. 97*	5	15 each arm	30 sec	at least 16k for men, 12k for women
7	All	Tire Jump *p. 112*	3	30 sec	30 sec	

LEVEL		MOVEMENT	SETS	REPS/TIME/INTERVAL	REST	COMMENTS
1	All	Inverted Row *p. 52*	2	15	30 sec	
2	All	H2H KB Swing *p. 61*	3	30 sec	30 sec	
3	All	Mountain Climbers *p. 114*	1	20		
4	All	Goblet Squat *p. 101*	3	30 sec	30 sec	KB/DB
5	All	Floor Wiper *p. 87*	1	25		max weight; up to 135lb for men, 95lb for women
6	All	Overhead Squat *p. 105*	1	10 each side		KB/DB
7	All	Tire Flip *p. 112*	3	50 ft	1 min	

LEVEL		MOVEMENT	SETS	REPS/TIME/INTERVAL	REST	COMMENTS
1	All	Static Hold: Chin over Bar *p. 49*	1	ALAP		
2	All	Deadlift *p. 55*	5	3	3 min	80% of 1RM
3	1	Up Dog into Down Dog *p. 141*	3	30 sec	30 sec	
	2 & 3	Up Dog into Down Dog *p. 141*	5	30 sec	30 sec	
4	All	RFESS *p. 84*	4	20 sec	20 sec	
5	All	Unicycle *p. 96*	3	30 sec/side	30 sec *after* 2nd side	
6	All	Dead Clean & Press *p. 97*	1	15 each side		16k for men, 8k–12k for women
7	All	Bench Press *p. 89*	5	10	90 sec	75% of 1RM

LEVEL		MOVEMENT	SETS	REPS/TIME/INTERVAL	REST	COMMENTS
1	All	Pull-Up *p. 47*	1	AMRAP	3–4 min *after* completing the set	
		Static Hold: Chin Over Bar *p. 49*	1	ALAP	2 min	
		Dead Hang from Midpoint *p. 49*	1	ALAP		
2	All	Deadlift *p. 55*	1	30		40% of 1RM
3	All	Push-Up *p. 67*	1	AMRAP		
4	All	Jump Squat *p. 81*	5	30 sec	30 sec	
5	All	Static Hold *p. 89*	1	ALAP		1RM weight
		Russian Twist *p. 96*	5	30 sec	30 sec	
6	All	Dead Clean *p. 97*	1	10 each side		moderate weight; move quickly
		Press *p. 97*	1	10 each side		moderate weight (12k or 16k); move quickly
7	All	Band Row *p. 119*	5	40	20 sec	

| 1 PULL-UP | 2 DEADLIFT | 3 PUSH-UP | 4 BOX JUMP | 5 FLOOR WIPER | 6 DEAD CLEAN & PRESS | 7 FINISHER |

	LEVEL	MOVEMENT	SETS	REPS/TIME/INTERVAL	REST	COMMENTS
1	All	Inverted Row p. 52	1	10		
2	All	Deadlift p. 55	1	50	as needed	135lb for men, 95lb for women
3	All	Push-Up p. 67	1	half your max		
4	All	Bodyweight Squat p. 100	1	10		
5	All	*Circuit:* Plank p. 93/ Bird Dog p. 94/High Plank p. 93	3	1 min each plank	1 min *after* each set	
6	All	Press p. 97	5	10 each side	45 sec	
7	All	Mountain Climbers p. 114	5	30 sec	30 sec	

	LEVEL	MOVEMENT	SETS	REPS/TIME/INTERVAL	REST	COMMENTS
1	All	Renegade Row p. 74	3	20 alternating arms	30 sec	KB/DB
2	All	*Circuit:* 2-Hand KB Swing p. 59/Right 1-Hand Swing/ Left 1-Hand Swing p. 60/ H2H KB Swing p. 61	3	30 sec each swing	1 min rest *after* working for 2 min	
3	1	Push-Up p. 67	5	10	1 min	
	2 & 3	Decline Push-Up p. 77	3	10	1 min	rest 3 min after last set
		Circuit: Walking Push-Up p. 71/ Up Dog into Down Dog p. 141	3	30 sec each		no rest between sets
4	All	Step-Up p. 85	1	10 each side		use 10lb weight vest or 2 light KB/DB
5	All	Leg Raise p. 92	3	10	1 min	
6	All	Dead Clean p. 97	5	5 each side	1 min	heavy weight
7	All	Tire Flip with Jump p. 112	3	1 min	30 sec	flip tire once, jump in/out, flip again, etc.

	LEVEL	MOVEMENT	SETS	REPS/TIME/INTERVAL	REST	COMMENTS
1	All	Pull-Up p. 47	3	AMRAP	1 min	
2	All	1-Hand KB Swing p. 60	5	30 sec/side	30 sec	light weight
3	All	Triangle Push-Up p. 77	2	10 or your max	30 sec	
4	All	Box Jump p. 79	1	50	as needed	AQAP; shoot for 15 to 20 reps before rest
	All	Leg Thrust p. 92	1	10		
5	All	Press p. 97	4	30 sec/side	30 sec	light weight; slow
6 7	All	*Circuit:* Farmer's Walk p. 118/ Rack Walk Side 1/Rack Walk Side 2 p. 118/Overhead Static Hold Walk p. 121	3	30 sec each walk	1 min *after* each set	

	LEVEL	MOVEMENT	SETS	REPS/TIME/INTERVAL	REST	COMMENTS
1	All	Band Row *p. 119*	3	25	30 sec	both arms simultaneously; use heavy band
2	All	Deadlift *p. 55*	10	5	1 min	75–85% of 1RM
3	All	Band Push-Up *p. 119*	3	30 sec	30 sec	
4	All	Bodyweight Squat *p. 100*	1	25		
5	All	Floor Wiper *p. 87*	1	30		max static weight, or 135lb for men, 95lb for women
6	All	Windmill *p. 108*	1	10 each side	30 sec	moderate weight
7	All	Low Windmill *p. 108*	3	5 each side	30 sec	

	LEVEL	MOVEMENT	SETS	REPS/TIME/INTERVAL	REST	COMMENTS
1	All	1-Arm Supported Row *p. 53*	2	10 each side	30 sec	heavy weight
2	All	High Pull *p. 66*		10/12/14/16/18/20/10	rest the time it took to do both arms	
3	1	Up Dog into Down Dog *p. 141*	3	10	30 sec	
	2 & 3	Up Dog into Down Dog *p. 141*	5	10	30 sec	
4	All	Step-Up with Backward Lunge *p. 85*	5	10 each side	1 min	can add a weight vest or hold a KB at chest level
5	All	Plank *p. 93*	1	2 min		
6	All	Dead Clean & Press *p. 97*	5	40 sec	20 sec *after* each arm	
7	All	Sandbag Shoulder *p. 99*	3	10 each side		

	LEVEL	MOVEMENT	SETS	REPS/TIME/INTERVAL	REST	COMMENTS
1	All	Pull-Up *p. 47*	1	25		break up into manageable sets
2	All	Deadlift *p. 55*	1	50		men 135lb, women 95lb, break up into manageable sets
3	All	Push-Up *p. 67*	1	50		break up into manageable sets
4	All	Box Jump *p. 79*	1	50		break up into manageable sets
5	All	Floor Wiper *p. 87*	1	50		break up into manageable sets
6	All	Dead Clean & Press *p. 97*	1	25 each side		break up into manageable sets
1	All	Pull-Up *p. 47*	1	25		break up into manageable sets

1 PULL-UP	**2** DEADLIFT	**3** PUSH-UP	**4** BOX JUMP	**5** FLOOR WIPER	**6** DEAD CLEAN & PRESS	**7** FINISHER

	LEVEL	MOVEMENT	SETS	REPS/TIME/INTERVAL	REST	COMMENTS
1	All	Pull-Up p. 47	5	5	30 sec	
2	All	Suitcase Deadlift p. 63	5	10	15 sec	70% of 1RM; AQAP
3	1	Incline p. 78 or Standard p. 67	5	10	30 sec	
	2	Standard p. 67 or Decline p. 77	5	10	30 sec	
	3	Decline p. 77 or Band p. 119	5	10	30 sec	
4	All	Static Lunge p. 83	5	45 sec	30 sec *after* 2nd side	
5	All	Leg Thrust p. 92	5	10	15 sec	
	All	Bench Press p. 89	5	15	15 sec	men 135lb, women 95lb or 80% of 1RM, whichever is lighter
6	All	Overhead Squat p. 105	5	10 each side	30 sec	
7	All	Tire Flip p. 112	3	100 ft	1 min	
	All	Sled Push p. 115	3	100 ft	1 min	moderate weight, go fast

	LEVEL	MOVEMENT	SETS	REPS/TIME/INTERVAL	REST	COMMENTS
1	All	Pull-Up p. 47				If Day 13 was easy, add 1 rep per min. If not, stay with same number reps/min.
2	All	*Circuit:* 2-Hand KB Swing p. 59/ Right 1-Hand Swing/Left 1-Hand Swing p. 60/H2H KB Swing p. 61	5	30 sec of each swing	1 min *after* working for 2 min	
3	All	Walking Push-Up p. 71	5	30 sec	30 sec	
4	All	Jump Tuck p. 82	3	30 sec	15 sec	
5	All	Unicycle p. 96	3	30 sec/side	30 sec	
6	All	Windmill p. 108	3	1 min/side	30 sec	
7	All	Sled Pull p. 115	5	75 ft		moderate weight, sprint

	LEVEL	MOVEMENT	SETS	REPS/TIME/INTERVAL	REST	COMMENTS
1	All	Negative Pull-Up p. 47	1	AMRAP		
2	All	Deadlift p. 55	5	5	1 min	85% of 1RM
3	1	Density Push-Up p. 67		5 per min on the min		20 min total
	2	Density Push-Up p. 67		10 per min on the min		10 min total
	3	Density Push-Up p. 67		15 per min on the min		8 min total
4	All	Jumping Lunge p. 86	8	20 sec	10 sec	
5	All	Ab Rollout p. 121	3	AMRAP	30 sec	
6	All	Dead Clean p. 97	5	5	30 sec	heavy as possible
	All	Press p. 97	5	5	45 sec	heavy as possible
7	All	Sledgehammer p. 113	1	100 alternating sides		

	LEVEL	MOVEMENT	SETS	REPS/TIME/INTERVAL	REST	COMMENTS
1	All	Inverted Row *p. 52*	1	15		
2	All	Band Deadlift *p. 120*	3	10	15 sec	
3	All	Push-Up *p. 67*	1	AMRAP		
4	All	Step-Up *p. 85*	1	10 each side		
5	All	Floor Wiper *p. 87*	5	10	15 sec	
6	All	Press *p. 97*	1	10 each side		men 16k, women 8 or 12k
7	All	Unicycle *p. 96*	8	20 sec/side	10 sec	
		Sled Push *p. 115*	1	250 ft		light and fast

TEST DAY: DAY 30

	LEVEL	MOVEMENT	SETS	REPS/TIME/INTERVAL	REST	COMMENTS
1	All	Pull-Up *p. 47*	1	25		break up into manageable sets
2	All	Deadlift *p. 55*	1	50		men 135lb, women 95lb, break up into manageable sets
3	All	Push-Up *p. 67*	1	50		break up into manageable sets
4	All	Box Jump *p. 79*	1	50		break up into manageable sets
5	All	Floor Wiper *p. 87*	1	50		break up into manageable sets
6	All	Dead Clean & Press *p. 97*	1	25 each side		break up into manageable sets
1	All	Pull-Up *p. 47*	1	25		break up into manageable sets

| 1 PULL-UP | 2 DEADLIFT | 3 PUSH-UP | 4 BOX JUMP | 5 FLOOR WIPER | 6 DEAD CLEAN & PRESS | 7 FINISHER |

	LEVEL	MOVEMENT	SETS	REPS/TIME/INTERVAL	REST	COMMENTS
1	1	Pull-Up p. 47	20	3	20 min	supported if necessary
	2 & 3	Pull-Up p. 47	20	5	20 min	if you started with Level 1, use the same time/reps/sets you used at the end of Level 1
2	All	Deadlift p. 55	20	3	20 min	60% of 1RM; use same reps per min as Pull-Ups above
3	All	*Push-Up p. 67	2	10	1 min	incline if necessary
4	All	*Jump Tuck p. 82	2	10	1 min	
5	All	*KB Floor Press p. 91	2	10	30 sec	pair of bells should total or come close to 75% of bench press 1RM
6	All	*Press p. 97	2	10 each side	30 sec	men 16k, women 8 or 12k
	*Optional Circuit: Do starred exercises as noted above but no rest between exercises, 1 min max between rounds; 3 rounds total					
7	All	Sledgehammer p. 113	5	30 sec/side	30 sec after 2nd side	

	LEVEL	MOVEMENT	SETS	REPS/TIME/INTERVAL	REST	COMMENTS
1	All	REST				
2	All	REST				
3	All	Push-Up p. 67		10/9/8/7/6/5/4/3/2/1	minimal	stand up in between rungs; if these are easy, add weight vest
4	All	Forward Lunge p. 83	3	30 sec alternating legs	30 sec	beginner: body weight only; others use 2 bells: men 16k, women 12k
5	All	Floor Wiper p. 87	3	10	30 sec	use whichever is heavier: men 135lb, women 95lb or 90% of bench press 1RM
6	All	Dead Clean p. 97	3	10 each side	30 sec	heavy weight
7	All	Tire Flip p. 112	3	10	1 min	

	LEVEL	MOVEMENT	SETS	REPS/TIME/INTERVAL	REST	COMMENTS
1	All	Inverted or Ring Row p. 52	3	10	30 sec	
2	All	2-Hand KB Swing p. 59	5	40 sec	20 sec	men 24k, women 16k
3	All	REST				
4	All	Box Jump p. 79	5	10	30 sec	men: 24" box or as close as you can get women: 18" box or as close as you can get
5	All	REST				
6	All	Dead Clean & Press p. 97	5	10 each side	30 sec	men 16k, women 8 or 12k
7	All	Ab Rollout p. 121 or Walkout p. 134	3	AMRAP	30 sec	

	LEVEL	MOVEMENT	SETS	REPS/TIME/INTERVAL	REST	COMMENTS
1	All	Renegade Row *p. 74*	5	20 alternating arms	30 sec	men 16k, women 12k
2	All	1-Leg Deadlift *p. 62*	5	30 sec/side	30 sec	1 KB/DB; men 24k, women 12k
3	All	Triangle Push-Up *p. 77*	3	10	30 sec	
4	All	REST				
5	All	Unicycle *p. 96*	3	30 sec/side	30 sec *after* 2nd side	
6	All	REST				
7	All	Sled Pull *p. 115*	3	100 ft	1 min	light weight; sprint with it
		Burpees *pp. 116–17*	5	30 sec	30 sec	

	LEVEL	MOVEMENT	SETS	REPS/TIME/INTERVAL	REST	COMMENTS
1	All	Density Pull-Up *p. 47*	20	20 min		Use same time/rep you did on Day 1. If it was easy, up the reps per min by 1.
2	All	Density Deadlift *p. 55*	20	20 min		Use same time/rep/weight you did on Day 1. If it was easy, add 1 rep or add 10lb to the bar, or both.
3	1	*Standard *p. 67* or Incline *p. 78*	3	10	30 sec	
	2 & 3	*Decline Push-Up *p. 77*	3	10	30 sec	
4	All	*RFESS *p. 84*	3	10 each side	30 sec	2 moderate KB/DB
5	All	*Low Windmill *p. 108*	3	10 each side	30 sec	heavy weight; minimum 24k men, 16k women
6	All	*Dead Clean *p. 97*	3	30 sec alternating arms	30 sec	2 bells: men 16k, women 12 or 18k
		Optional Circuit: Do starred exercises for 30 sec each (30 sec each side where applicable, no rest between sides); 15 sec rest between exercises; 5 rounds total				
7	All	Sled Push *p. 115*	3	100 ft	1 min	heavy weight
		Burpees *pp. 116–17*	5	30 sec	30 sec	

	LEVEL	MOVEMENT	SETS	REPS/TIME/INTERVAL	REST	COMMENTS
1	All	REST				
2	All	REST				
3	All	Push-Up *p. 67*		1/2/3/4/5/6/7/8/9/10	pause briefly between rungs	beginners do inclines or from knees; advanced use weight vest
4	All	*Goblet Squat *p. 101*	3	10	30 sec	minimum 24k men, 16k women
5	All	Floor Wiper *p. 87*	3	10	30 sec	use whichever is heavier: men 135lb, women 95lb or 80% of bench press 1RM
6	All	*Press *p. 97*	3	15 each side	30 sec	light & fast
7	All	*Sandbag Shoulder *p. 99*	5	30 sec	30 sec	alternate sides each rep
		Optional Circuit: Do starred exercises for 30 sec each (30 sec each side where applicable, no rest between sides); 30 sec rest between exercises; 5 rounds total				

1 PULL-UP   **2** DEADLIFT   **3** PUSH-UP   **4** BOX JUMP   **5** FLOOR WIPER   **6** DEAD CLEAN & PRESS   **7** FINISHER

	LEVEL	MOVEMENT	SETS	REPS/TIME/INTERVAL	REST	COMMENTS
1	All	*Static Hold: Chin over Bar p. 49	1	ALAP		advanced: use weight vest
2	All	*Suitcase Deadlift p. 63	5	5	30 sec	2 heavy bells
3	All	REST				
4	All	Box Jump p. 79	5	10	30 sec	men 24" box, women 18" box
5	All	REST				
6	All	Dead Clean & Press p. 97	5	10 each side	30 sec	men 16k, women 8 or 12k
7	All	*Sledgehammer p. 113	5	30 sec/side	30 sec *after* 2nd side	

*Optional Circuit: Do Static Hold and Suitcase Deadlift for 1 min each and Sledgehammer for 30 sec each arm; 30 sec rest between exercises; 5 rounds total

	LEVEL	MOVEMENT	SETS	REPS/TIME/INTERVAL	REST	COMMENTS
1	All	High Pull p. 66	3	30 sec/side	30 sec	
2	All	2-Hand KB Swing p. 59	1	1 min		light weight
3	All	Walking Push-Up p. 71	3	30 sec	30 sec	if doing knee push-ups, try to stay off them while walking over to the other side
4	All	REST				
5	All	KB Floor Press p. 91	2	15	30 sec	2 KB/DB at 75% of bench press 1RM
6	All	REST				
7	All	Tire Flip p. 112	3	12	30 sec	move quickly

	LEVEL	MOVEMENT	SETS	REPS/TIME/INTERVAL	REST	COMMENTS
1	All	Density Pull-Up p. 47	20	20 min		Use same time/rep scheme you did on Day 1. If it was easy, up the reps per min by 1.
2	All	Density Deadlift p. 55	20	20 min		Use same time/reps/weight you did on Day 1. If it was easy, add 1 rep or 10lb to the bar, or both.
3	1	*Incline Push-Up p. 78	2	12	45 sec	
	2	*Standard p. 67 or Decline Push-Up p. 77	2	12	45 sec	
	3	*Decline Push-Up p.77 or with Weight Vest p. 90	2	12	45 sec	
4	All	*Jump Tuck p. 82	2	12	45 sec	
5	All	*Leg Thrust p. 92	1	20		
6	All	*KB Floor Press p. 91	2	12	45 sec	men 16k, women 8 or 12k

*Optional Circuit: Do starred exercises for 20 sec each (for KB Floor Press, switch arms each round); 10 sec rest between exercises; 8 rounds total

	LEVEL	MOVEMENT	SETS	REPS/TIME/INTERVAL	REST	COMMENTS
7	All	Ab Rollout p. 121 or Walkout p. 134	5	AMRAP	30 sec	

	LEVEL	MOVEMENT	SETS	REPS/TIME/INTERVAL	REST	COMMENTS
1	All	REST				
2	All	REST				
3	All	Push-Up *p. 67*		11/10/9/8/7/6/5/4/3/2/1	minimal	
4	All	Forward Lunge *p. 83*	3	30 sec alternating sides	30 sec	2 light KB/DB hanging down
5	All	Floor Wiper *p. 87*	3	12	30 sec	use whichever is greater: men 135lb, women 95lb or 75% of 1RM
6	All	Dead Clean *p. 97*	5	30 sec	30 sec	heavy weight
7	All	Sled Pull *p. 115*	4	100 ft	45 sec	moderate weight; move quickly
		Burpees *pp. 116–17*	5	30 sec	30 sec	

	LEVEL	MOVEMENT	SETS	REPS/TIME/INTERVAL	REST	COMMENTS
1	All	Inverted or Ring Row *p. 52*	2	15	45 sec	
2	All	2-Hand KB Swing *p. 59*	5	50 sec	10 sec	light to moderate weight
3	All	REST				
4	All	Box Jump *p. 79*	5	12	30 sec	men: 24" or as close as possible; women: 18" or as close as possible; complete AQAP
5	All	REST				
6	All	Dead Clean & Press *p. 97*	5	12	30 sec	men 16k, women 8 or 12k; complete AQAP
7	All	Sled Push *p. 115*	3	100 ft	45 sec	heavy weight
		Mountain Climbers *p. 114*	5	30 sec	30 sec	

	LEVEL	MOVEMENT	SETS	REPS/TIME/INTERVAL	REST	COMMENTS
1	All	*Renegade Row *p. 74*	5	24 alternating sides	30 sec	
2	All	*1-Leg Deadlift *p. 62*	5	30 sec	30 sec *after* 2nd side	
3	All	*Triangle Push-Up *p. 77*	3	12	30 sec	
4	All	REST				
5	All	*Unicycle *p. 96*	4	30 sec/side	30 sec *after* 2nd side	
6	All	REST				
7	All	*Sandbag Shoulder *p. 99*	5	30 sec	30 sec	alternate sides

Optional Circuit: Do starred exercises for 40 sec each (40 sec each side where applicable, no rest between sides; *but* alternate sides for Renegade Rows and Sandbag Shoulder); 20 sec rest between exercises; 5 rounds total

| 1 | PULL-UP | 2 | DEADLIFT | 3 | PUSH-UP | 4 | BOX JUMP | 5 | FLOOR WIPER | 6 | DEAD CLEAN & PRESS | 7 | FINISHER |

ALL LEVELS—Rest Day: do tai chi, walk, gardening, etc.

LEVEL		MOVEMENT	SETS	REPS/TIME/INTERVAL	REST	COMMENTS
1	All	Pull-Up p. 47	25	AQAP	minimal	do in chunks
2	All	Deadlift p. 55	50	AQAP	minimal	men 135lb, women 95lb
3	All	Push-Up p. 67	50	AQAP	minimal	do in chunks
4	All	Box Jump p. 79	50	AQAP	minimal	men 24" box, women 18" box
5	All	Floor Wiper p. 87	50	AQAP	minimal	men 135lb, women 95lb
6	All	Dead Clean & Press p. 97	25 each side	AQAP	minimal	men 16k, women 8 or 12k
1	All	Pull-Up p. 47	25	AQAP	minimal	do in chunks

ALL LEVELS—Rest Day: do tai chi, walk, gardening, etc.

LEVEL		MOVEMENT	SETS	REPS/TIME/INTERVAL	REST	COMMENTS
1	All	Density Pull-Up p. 47	20	20 min		Use same time/rep scheme you did on Day 1. If it was easy, up the reps per min by 1.
2	All	Density Deadlift p. 55	20	20 min		Use same time/reps/weight you did on Day 1. If it was easy, add 1 rep or 10lb to the bar, or both.
3	1	*Incline p. 78 or Standard Push-Up p. 67	3	12	45 sec	
	2	*Standard p. 67 or Decline Push-Up p. 77	3	12	45 sec	
	3	*Decline p. 77 or add Weight Vest p. 90	3	12	45 sec	
4	All	*RFESS p. 84	3	15	30 sec	2 moderate KB/DB hanging down
5	All	*Low Windmill p. 108	3	12 each side	30 sec	heavy weight
6	All	*Dead Clean p. 97	4	30 sec/side	30 sec	one pair; men 16k, women 8 or 12k
		*Optional Circuit: Do starred exercises for 30 sec each (30 sec each side where applicable, no rest between sides); 30 sec rest between exercises; 4 rounds total				
7	All	Band Row p. 119	3	40 sec	20 sec	
		Farmer's Walk p. 118	3	100 ft	30 sec	

LEVEL		MOVEMENT	SETS	REPS/TIME/INTERVAL	REST	COMMENTS
1	All	REST				
2	All	REST				
3	All	Push-Up *p. 67*		1/2/3/4/5/6/7/8/9/10/11	minimal	
4	All	Step-Up *p. 85*	2	10 each side	30 sec	use same box you jump to
5	All	Floor Wiper *p. 87*	3	15	30 sec	men 135lb, women 95lb; or 95% of 1RM
6	All	Overhead Windmill *p. 109*	3	5 each side	30 sec	moderate weight
7	All	Mountain Climbers *p. 114*	8	20 sec	10 sec	rest 30 sec before moving on to next exercise
		Dead Clean *p. 97*	8	20 sec/arm	10 sec	rest 30 sec before moving on to next exercise
		High Pull *p. 66*	8	20 sec	10 sec	switch hands each interval

LEVEL		MOVEMENT	SETS	REPS/TIME/INTERVAL	REST	COMMENTS
1	All	Static Hold: Chin over Bar *p. 49*	1	ALAP		
2	All	Suitcase Deadlift *p. 63*	5	5	1 min	2 heavy DB/KB
3	All	REST				
4	All	Box Jump *p. 79*	5	15	minimal	men 24", women 18"
5	All	REST				
6	All	Dead Clean & Press *p. 97*	4	15	30 sec	men 16k, women 8 or 12k
7	All	Sled Pull *p. 115*	4	100 ft	1 min	heavy weight, but try to move quickly
		Burpees *pp. 116–17*	5	30 sec	30 sec	

LEVEL		MOVEMENT	SETS	REPS/TIME/INTERVAL	REST	COMMENTS
1	All	High Pull *p. 66*	4	30 sec	30 sec	
2	All	2-Hand KB Swing *p. 59*	3	1 min	30 sec	moderate weight
3	1	Push-Up *p. 67*	5	10	20 sec	
	2	Decline Push-Up *p. 77*	5	10	20 sec	
	3	Walking Push-Up *p. 71*	5	10	30 sec	
4	All	REST				
5	All	Leg Thrust *p. 92*	1	25	2 min *after* each set	
		Barbell Floor Press *p. 91*	5	3	1 min	95% of bench press 1RM
6	All	REST				
7	All	Double Windmill *p. 109*	3	8 each side	30 sec	use lighter bell overhead and slightly heavier bell off the floor

1 PULL-UP   2 DEADLIFT   3 PUSH-UP   4 BOX JUMP   5 FLOOR WIPER   6 DEAD CLEAN & PRESS   7 FINISHER

	LEVEL	MOVEMENT	SETS	REPS/TIME/INTERVAL	REST	COMMENTS
1	All	Density Pull-Up *p. 47*	20	20 min		If last attempt at these was easy, add another rep per min.
2	All	Density Deadlift *p. 55*	20	20 min		If last attempt at these was easy, add another rep per min.
3	All	Triangle Push-Up *p. 77*	1	15		
4	All	Jump Squat *p. 81*	4	15	30 sec	
5	All	Renegade Row *p. 74*	3	20 alternating arms	30 sec	
6	All	Dead Clean *p. 97*	5	10 each side	45 sec	men 24k or more, women 16k or more
		Push Press *p. 97*	5	10 each side	30 sec	heavier than your usual press weight, or men 24k, women 16k
7	All	Sledgehammer *p. 113*	5	40 sec alternating sides	20 sec	
		Tire Flip *p. 112*	1	100 ft		

	LEVEL	MOVEMENT	SETS	REPS/TIME/INTERVAL	REST	COMMENTS
1	All	REST				
2	All	REST				
3	All	Push-Up *p. 67*		11/10/9/8/7/6/5/4/3/2/1		beginners: avoid knees
4	All	Backward Lunge *p. 83*	5	30 sec alternating legs	30 sec	
5	All	Floor Wiper *p. 87*	4	15	30 sec	men 135lb, women 95lb
6	All	Overhead Squat *p. 105*	1	10 each side		men 16k, women 8 or 12k
7	All	*Circuit:* High Plank *p. 93*/ Sandbag Shoulder *p. 99*/ Ab Rollout *p. 121* or Walkout *p. 134*	5	30 sec each item	30 sec *after* each set	

	LEVEL	MOVEMENT	SETS	REPS/TIME/INTERVAL	REST	COMMENTS
1	All	Negative Pull-Up *p. 47*	5	10	1 min	
2	All	*Circuit*: 2-Hand KB Swing *p. 59*/Left 1-Hand KB Swing/ Right 1-Hand KB Swing *p. 60*/ H2H KB Swing *p. 61*	5	30 sec each swing	1 min *after* each set	
3	All	REST				
4	All	Jump Tuck *p. 82*	2	15	30 sec	rest 2 min before starting next exercise
	All	Step-Up with Lunge *p. 85*	3	20 alternating legs	1 min	use same box you usually jump to; add sandbag
5	All	REST				
6	All	Dead Clean & Press *p. 97*	3	20 each side	30 sec	men 16k, women 8 or 10k
	All	Overhead Squat *p. 105*	5	5 each side	30 sec	moderate weight: minimum 20k men, 12k women
7	All	*Circuit*: Squat Thrust *p. 136*/ Shuffles *p. 136*/Mountain Climbers *p. 137*/Jumping Jacks *p. 137*	3	30 sec each item	30 sec *after* each set	

	LEVEL	MOVEMENT	SETS	REPS/TIME/INTERVAL	REST	COMMENTS
1	All	*Inverted or Ring Row *p. 52*	4	15	20 sec	
2	All	*1-Leg Deadlift *p. 62*	5	30 sec	30 sec	
3	All	*Wide Push-Up *p. 78*	2	15	30 sec to 1 min	beginners, avoid knees
4	All	REST				
5	All	*Russian Twist *p. 96*	5	40 sec	20 sec	
	All	*KB Floor Press *p. 91*	8	20 sec	10 sec	
6	All	REST				
		*Optional Circuit: Do starred exercises for 30 sec each (30 sec each side where applicable, no rest between sides); 15 sec rest between exercises; 3 rounds total				
7	All	*Circuit*: Tire Flip *p. 112*/ Jump Squat *p. 104*/Walking Push-Up *p. 71*/High Pull (alternating arms) *p. 66*	3	Tire Flip 50 ft; 30 sec each for everything else	1 min *after* each set	

1 PULL-UP **2** DEADLIFT **3** PUSH-UP **4** BOX JUMP **5** FLOOR WIPER **6** DEAD CLEAN & PRESS **7** FINISHER

	LEVEL	MOVEMENT	SETS	REPS/TIME/INTERVAL	REST	COMMENTS
1	All	Pull-Up p. 47		25		AQAP; do in chunks
2	All	Deadlift p. 55	10	5	1 min	85% of 1RM
3	1	*Incline p. 78 or Standard Push-Up p. 67	2	10	20 sec	
	2	*Standard p. 67 or Decline Push-Up p. 77	2	10	20 sec	
	3	*Decline Push-Up p. 77	2	10	20 sec	if easy, add weight vest
4	All	*RFESS p. 84	3	10 each side	30 sec	2 KB/DB hanging down; men 16k, women 12k
5	All	*Low Windmill p. 108	2	8 each side	30 sec	men 24k, women 16k
6	All	*Sandbag Clean to Press p. 106	3	8	1 min	heavy weight: minimum 50lb men (70 preferably), 25lb women (35 preferably)

*Optional Circuit: Do starred exercises for 30 sec each (30 sec each side where applicable, no rest between sides, *but* alternate sides for Sandbag Clean to Press); 30 sec rest between exercises; 4 rounds total

	LEVEL	MOVEMENT	SETS	REPS/TIME/INTERVAL	REST	COMMENTS
7	All	Inverted or Ring Row p. 52	5	10	1 min	use weight vest if you're strong enough
		Sled Push p. 115	2	100 ft	1 min	go heavy

	LEVEL	MOVEMENT	SETS	REPS/TIME/INTERVAL	REST	COMMENTS
1	All	REST				
2	All	REST				
3	All	Push-Up p. 67		50		AQAP; do in chunks
4	All	Goblet Squat p. 101	3	12	30 sec	men 24k, women 16k
5	All	Floor Wiper p. 87	4	15	20 sec	men 135lb, women 95lb
6	All	Press p. 97	3	15	30 sec	men 12k, women 8k
7	All	Bench Press p. 89	3	10	20 sec	50% of 1RM; move quickly
		Mountain Climbers p. 114	4	30 sec	15 sec	

	LEVEL	MOVEMENT	SETS	REPS/TIME/INTERVAL	REST	COMMENTS
1	All	Inverted or Ring Row *p. 52*	1	10		
2	All	Double KB Swing *p. 59*	5	10	30 sec	heavy weight (minimum): men 2x16k, women 2x12k
3	All	REST				
4	All	Bodyweight Squat *p. 100*	8	20 sec	10 sec	Rest at bottom of squat. Rest 2 min before starting next exercise.
	1	Static Lunge *p. 83*	4	30 sec/side	30 sec	
	2 & 3	Jump Lunge *p. 86*	4	30 sec	30 sec	
5	All	REST				
6	All	Dead Clean *p. 97*	5	5 each side		heavy weight: minimum 24k men, 16k women
7	All	Band Row *p. 119*	3	40 sec	20 sec	
		Farmer's Walk *p. 118*	3	100 ft	1 min	2 KB/DB hanging down; minimum 24k men, 16k women

	LEVEL	MOVEMENT	SETS	REPS/TIME/INTERVAL	REST	COMMENTS
1	All	1-Arm Supported Row *p. 53*	2	5 each side	30 sec	heavy weight: men 24k, women 16k
2	All	High Pull *p. 66*		10/12/14/16/18/20/10	rest is the time it takes to complete each rung; no rest until you've done both arms	
3	All	Walking Push-Up *p. 71*	3	30 sec	30 sec	
4	All	REST				
5	All	Unicycle *p. 96*	5	30 sec/side	30 sec	
6	All	REST				
7	All	Ab Rollout p. *121* or Walkout p. *134*	5	AMRAP	30 sec	
		Tire Flip with Jump *p. 112*	3	15	1 min	flip tire once, jump in/out, flip again, etc.
		Mountain Climbers *p. 114*	8	20 sec	10 sec	rest in push-up position

| **1** PULL-UP | **2** DEADLIFT | **3** PUSH-UP | **4** BOX JUMP | **5** FLOOR WIPER | **6** DEAD CLEAN & PRESS | **7** FINISHER |

ALL LEVELS—Rest Day: do something different than your workout days, but easy

	LEVEL	MOVEMENT	SETS	REPS/TIME/INTERVAL	REST	COMMENTS
1	All	Pull-Up *p. 47*		25		AQAP, no kipping
2	All	Deadlift *p. 55*		50		men 135lb, women 95lb
3	All	Push-Up *p. 67*		50		Stay off your knees!
4	All	Box Jump *p. 79*		50		men 24", women 18"
5	All	Floor Wiper *p. 87*		50		men 135lb, women 95lb
6	All	Dead Clean & Press *p. 97*		25 each side		men 16k, women 8 or 12k
1	All	Pull-Up *p. 47*		25		AQAP, no kipping

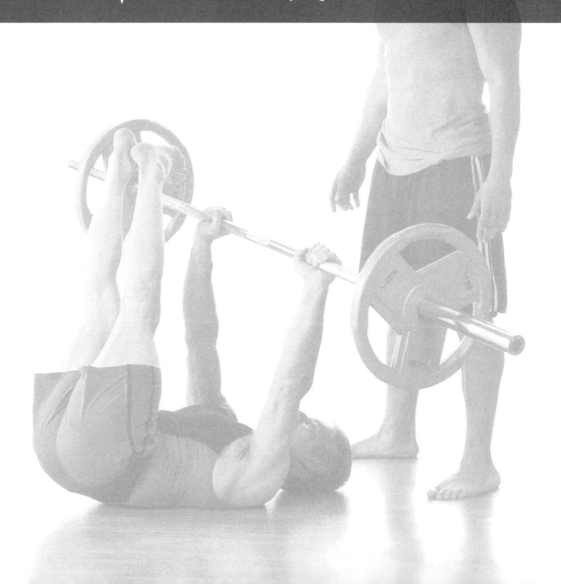

PART 3

The Exercises

Pull-Ups

The Spartan Warrior Workout calls for 50 dead-hang pull-ups, 25 at the beginning of the workout and 25 at the end. For most people, pull-ups are probably the most challenging of the exercises in this workout. They're a total-body exercise that requires serious back strength. The core is heavily involved and, surprisingly, so are the legs, even in a dead-hang pull-up. One major factor in the ability to do pull-ups is grip strength; if you can't hold your weight on the bar, you aren't going to be able to pull yourself up.

Many people struggle for years trying to do more than a few pull-ups and some never manage to get even one. Usually it's because they haven't been taught the proper way to do pull-ups and the progressions that create the strength needed to do them. See "Determining Your Current Level" on page 48 to see where you stand. Program 1 (pages 23–34) provides progressions to help you improve your pull-up ability.

TERMINOLOGY & BODY POSITION

Before we go on, let's make sure we're on the same page. A chin-up is done with the palms facing you as you're gripping the bar, while a pull-up is done with the palms facing away. Because chin-ups are mostly a biceps exercise, they're much easier to do than pull-ups.

One other distinction: We're only going to be working on the dead-hang pull-up, as opposed to kipping pull-ups. Dead-hang pull-ups start with the arms extended but with a slight bend in the elbows and the shoulders packed in tight (don't let them come out of the sockets). Kipping pull-ups involve swinging the legs and using momentum to get the chin over the bar or the chest to the bar, and people have come up with elaborate ways to create that momentum. While kipping certainly allows you to do more pull-ups, you're basically cheating. Kipping can also increase the risk of shoulder injury since the shoulders are what take the stress of the descent.

Your hands should be directly above your shoulders. You can go a little wider or narrower, whatever is more comfortable, but going too wide is very hard on the shoulders. Having your hands too close together makes doing a pull-up even harder.

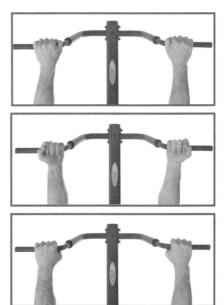

Top: Proper pull-up grip (false grip). Middle & bottom: Improper pull-up grips

Your grip should be a thumbless, or false, grip, meaning your thumb is over the bar with your fingers, not wrapped around the bar. You should be holding the bar at the base of the fingers, just before they go into the hand itself (as opposed to the middle of the palm).

THE MOVEMENT

1 Hang from the bar with your hands in line with your shoulders or slightly wider. Use a false grip, pack your shoulders in their sockets and allow your legs and elbows to be slightly bent (this keeps tension through the upper body).

2 Contract all the muscles in your body and pull your-self up, thinking about bringing your elbows to your sides and your chin over the bar so it's parallel to the floor. Don't let your elbows flare out to the sides.

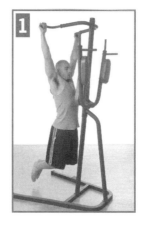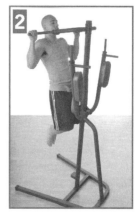

Lower yourself quickly but with control until you return to the starting position. Pause then repeat. There should be no bouncing out of the descent and no leg swing.

DETERMINING YOUR CURRENT LEVEL

Now that you know how to do a proper pull-up, try it and see how many you can do. Can you do more than 15? One? None? Use the chart to determine your level.

NUMBER OF PULL-UPS	LEVEL	DESCRIPTION
0–5	1	BEGINNER You'll need to start by doing supported pulling and static holds. Then you'll do pull-ups in small sets over different time frames, plus other exercises to augment the pull-ups.
5–10	2	INTERMEDIATE You can add a light weight while practicing the pull-up and do more intense practice.
10–15	3	INTERMEDIATE+ You're at the point where adding a bit more weight while you practice and then doing the same assistance movements as in Level 1 and 2 will get you over 15 reps
15+	4	ADVANCED You can probably do one-arm pull-ups, which are be-yond the scope of this book. Keep doing what you've been doing and focus on the exercises in this workout that you're weak in.

VARIATIONS & SUPPLEMENTAL EXERCISES

No matter what your level, the following variations and supplemental exercises will help improve your pull-up numbers. For instance, the rowing movement uses a lot of the same upper- and mid-back muscles as the pull-up so using them as assistance work will make your pull-ups stronger.

If you're at the beginner level, only able to do a few or maybe even none at all right now, these will be your primary focus until you can do one or two pull-ups. These progressions will improve the strength of the lats, deltoids, rhomboids, trapezius, hands, forearms and other muscles involved in performing pull-ups.

DEAD HANG

This is the starting position for the pull-up. Simply holding onto the bar for many people, especially women, is tough. Grip strength is the limiting factor.

1 Get on a bar (hands directly in line with your shoulders or slightly wider) and hang with your elbows almost straight and knees bent 90 degrees and crossed behind you (this helps keep stress off your lower back). See how long you can hang. If you can hang 30 seconds or more, your grip strength is good; if you can hang more than a minute, it's great. If you can't hold on for 30 seconds, then this is where you start—do holds for time, gradually increasing the hang time until you can hold it for at least one minute.

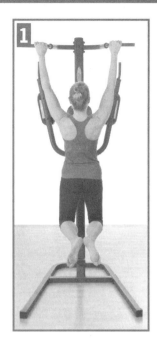

STATIC HOLD: CHIN OVER BAR

This will increase your strength very quickly.

1 With a partner or a high box, get your chin above the bar with no foot support and hang there as long as you can. Keep your entire body tense. Squeeze your abs, butt, thighs and everything else. When you can no longer maintain the hold, lower down as slowly as you can. Do this several times but not to failure. Practice this several times throughout the day and you will see results much more quickly.

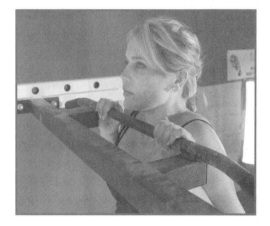

This reduces the amount of weight you're trying to move. Whatever you use for a foot rest needs to be at a height where, when your knees are straight, your chin is just over the bar.

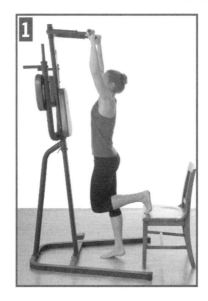

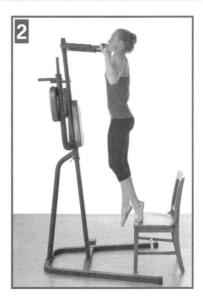

1–2 Position a bench or chair under the pull-up bar so that your feet can rest on it when you're in the dead hang. With your hands placed as described in the Dead Hang (page 49) and using a false grip, pull yourself up as high as you can. Use your feet as necessary, but as little as possible. Focus on bringing your elbows to your sides.

Slowly (count 1001, 1002, 1003) lower yourself until your arms are straight.

PROGRESSION: As you get stronger, move the support out in front of you so that when you're going up and down your lower back stays flat. Known as the jack-knife pull-up, this allows you to use your legs, but nowhere near as much as when your feet are under you.

VARIATION: If you're short and don't have a high enough support, pull up until your legs are straight even though you may not have your chin over the bar. You can also have a partner hold your feet.

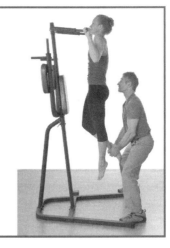

HALF PULL-UP

Pulling from the bottom, even only slightly, will strengthen the portion of the lats involved in the initial phase of a pull-up. Doing a partial negative from the top position, starting with the chin above the bar, strengthens the upper portion of the pull. As you get stronger at the top and bottom you'll find you're going halfway down and halfway up, which means you should be able to do a full pull-up. Once you can do one it's a matter of building muscular endurance.

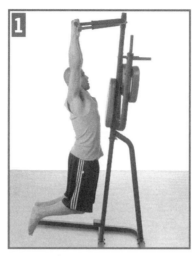 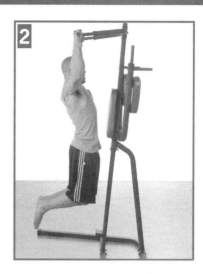

Lower Half

1-2 From the dead hang position, without foot support, pull hard, even if you only move an inch, then go back to dead hang. Do this as many times as possible but never going to failure; always keep one or two in the tank.

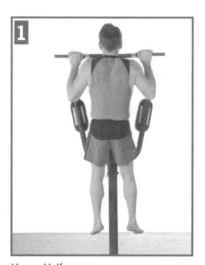 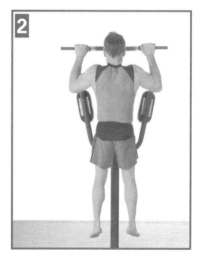

Upper Half

1-2 Get your chin above the bar and lower yourself a little then pull back up, gradually increasing the distance you travel. Stay tight!

JUMPING PULL-UP

1-2 Jump up from the floor or a box if necessary, getting your chin over the bar. You should not be able to reach the floor or your box from the dead hang position. Slowly lower yourself until your arms are straight then jump back up. Be careful, you can easily overdo these and get really sore.

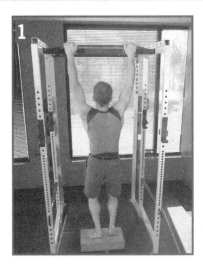 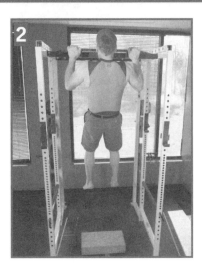

INVERTED ROW

These hit the pull-up muscles at different angles, which will stimulate them to get stronger because the load is different and will help you to progress more quickly.

1 Take a barbell and set it up so you can hang beneath it with your arms fully extended and torso parallel to the floor. Grab the bar with your hands about shoulder-width apart, palms facing away.

2 Pull your chest to the bar. Keep your elbows in, close to your body. Do as many as you can but not to failure.

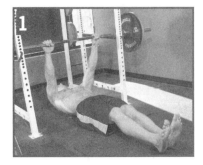 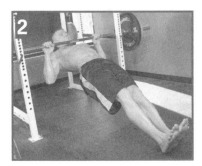

RINGS VARIATION: If you have access to gymnastics rings, you can perform inverted rows on them instead. They'll let you adjust the difficulty by changing your angle of inclination. The closer to parallel your body is to the floor, the harder the rows are. Try to keep your legs straight, but bend your knees slightly if you must.

ONE-ARM SUPPORTED ROW

If you have access to a rowing machine you can use that for rows. However, bent rows with a barbell stress the lower back, and the risk-to-benefit ratio isn't worth the risk of blowing out your back.

1 Place one leg forward and bend the knee, keeping the back leg straight and both feet firmly on the ground. Angle the back foot about 45 degrees. The kettlebell/dumbbell will be on the floor to the inside of your front foot, about even with the ball of the foot. Create a long spine by lifting your chest and pushing your hips back. Put your forearm across your thigh just above your knee (if your left leg is forward, your left forearm is on that leg).

2 With your right arm, pull up the bell with your lats, not your shoulder, and bring the weight toward your hip as though you were going to put it in your pocket. Keep your arm close to your body so that the inner part of your upper arm brushes your side; do not flare out your elbow. Move in a slow, controlled manner. Stay tight through the core—don't let your hips rotate or your torso move. Keep your chest out and maintain a flat back.

Lower the weight slowly back to the start position. If you're using a kettlebell and have a deep stance, you should be able to put it back on the floor, but don't worry if you can't.

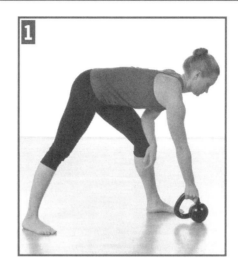

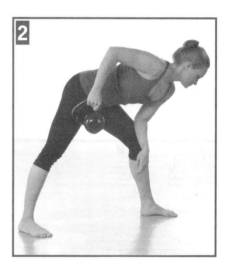

Doing planks will strengthen your core and teach you how to recruit as much tension in your body as possible for maximal strength.

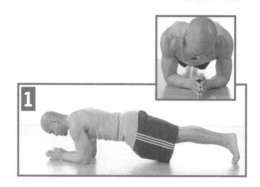

1 Place your forearms on the floor parallel to each other; align your elbows under your shoulders. You may keep your palms face down on the floor or place the outer edges of your hands/fists on the floor. Extend your legs behind you like you would for a push-up, keeping your hips in the same plane as your shoulders. Squeeze your abs, glutes, hamstrings, quads, arms—everything but your neck—and hold that position. Make sure your back is flat; don't let your back sag or your hips go high or low.

HIGH PLANK: Assume the top position of a push-up, placing your hands on the floor in line with your shoulders, keeping your back flat, your knees straight and your hips in the same plane as your shoulders. Squeeze everything and hold it for as long as you can.

ONE-ARM PLANK: From forearm or high plank, raise one arm and hold it straight out in front of you, as close to level with your back as possible. Do both sides.

ONE-LEG PLANK: Raise one foot, keeping the leg in the same plane as the body. Do both sides.

ONE-ARM/ONE-LEG PLANK: Raise the right arm and left leg, then switch sides.

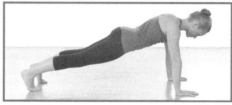

High Plank

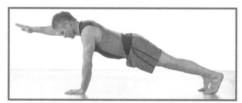

One-Arm Plank

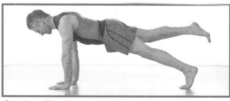

One-Leg Plank

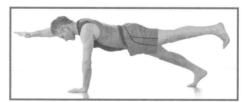

One-Arm/One-Leg Plank

Deadlift

The deadlift is one of the most powerful lifts around. It's also pretty straightforward: Pick a barbell off the floor and stand up. So what's so hard about that? Well, with light weights not much, but when you start going heavier, there are a lot of details that can make or break you. You'll soon see why proper form is required.

"Light" and "heavy" are relative terms, and the Spartan Warrior Workout calls for 50 deadlifts performed with a 135-pound barbell, including the weight of the bar, which is standardized at 45 pounds. Most guys should be able to do at least a few reps at this weight, but women may find it a bit tougher. So we'll scale this back for women and have them use 95 pounds instead.

First we'll break down the movement then determine your 1 RM (rep maximum). Once we've determined that, we'll craft a plan to improve the endurance of your glutes, hamstrings and lower back primarily so that you can begin to do 10 to 20 reps or more in a set. For the workout, you'll need to do the 50 deadlifts quickly; because there's a tendency to get sloppy, you must pay strict attention to form and make sure you rest when you need to so you don't get fatigued and injured.

BODY POSITION

There are several variations to the deadlift in regards to stance and grip. We'll be performing what is known as the *conventional deadlift*. This has the feet hip- to shoulder-width apart and the arms hanging straight down outside the legs. The *sumo deadlift*, named after the wide stance sumo wrestlers take, has the feet spread wider than the shoulder and the arms hanging inside the legs.

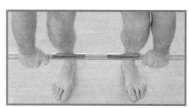

Double overhand grip

Hand placement on the bar should be such that the arms hang straight down from the shoulder blades and the hands are just out over the shins. The grip can be done one of two ways: with the hands wrapped over the bar (double overhand) or one hand over and one hand under the bar, which is typically referred to as an alternating grip.

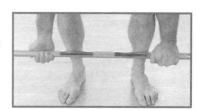

Alternating grip

THE MOVEMENT

1 Approach the bar with your feet hip-width or slightly wider apart. The bar should be over the mid-foot, about where your shoelaces are tied; it will be an inch or so from your shins.

2 Bend over at the waist, reach straight down and place your hands on the bar using the alternating grip. Your hands should be just outside your legs. Once you set your grip, push your knees forward until your shins touch the bar, then lift your chest up. Your lower back should be flat or slightly arched. Your shoulders will be in front of the bar but there should be a straight line from your scapulas to the bar. Looking at it from the side, a line drawn from your shoulder blade through your arm to the bar should be perfectly vertical.

3 To stand up, straighten your knees and move your hips forward. As the bar moves up past your knees, your torso comes up. Keep your arms straight throughout the lift; don't try to lift the bar with your arms by

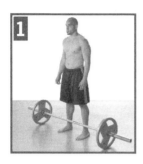 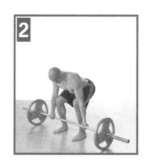 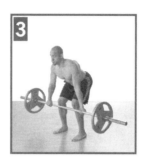 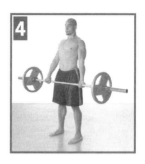

bending your elbows. As you stand, keep the bar in close—you should be literally pulling the bar up your shins and maintaining contact as it comes up your thighs. Also make sure not to straighten your knees before the bar is above them. If your knees straighten out too soon, your hips will come up too quickly, which can cause back issues.

4 At the top position standing fully upright, your glutes, hamstrings, quads, core and grip should be locked out. Everything should be tight even if the weight is light for you.

Typically, heavy deadlifts are dropped to the floor, but then you usually only do 1 rep with a short reset before the next rep. Since we need to do 50 reps, we have to learn to lower the weight quickly but with control. The eccentric or negative portion of the deadlift is pretty much the reverse of the concentric movement. Push your hips back, maintaining the same back angle you had on the ascent, and keep your knees straight. Keep your arms straight and your core tight. Once the bar has passed your knees, bend them while continuing to push your hips back. Keep your shins vertical. As with the ascent, the bar stays in contact with your thighs and shins all the way down.

As soon as the bar touches the floor, quickly reset your position, brace and stand back up. Maintain tension and proper skeletal alignment throughout the movement.

> ## THINGS TO WATCH FOR
>
> **Hips are too low**—if they come up first when your knees straighten, your hips were probably too low or the weight is too heavy.
>
> **Bar is not lined up with the scapulas**—the bar will swing out away from you.
>
> **Bar is not traveling in a vertical line**—your knees aren't straightening before your hips come up, or on the way down your knees are bending before the bar passes them.

DETERMINING YOUR 1 REP MAX (RM)

Determining the appropriate weight to use in the deadlift involves some experimentation. If you've never deadlifted before or only occasionally, follow the steps below to determine your 5 RM; from there we can estimate your 1 RM. If you've been deadlifting consistently for more than a few months, you should already have a good idea of what your 1 RM is and can skip this.

Use the table on the following page to figure your starting weight. *Note:* If you're not using training plates or are under 135 pounds total bar weight, elevate the bar so that it's 8.5 inches from the floor. This is the standard height when using two 45-pound plates on an Olympic bar.

EXPERIENCE LEVEL	WOMEN	MEN
Never deadlifted	45 lb. (empty bar)	95 lb.
Deadlifted a few times	65 lb.	115 lb.
Deadlifted consistently for few months	95 lb. or last session weight	135 lb. or last session weight
Deadlifted consistently for a year-plus	your last session weight	your last session weight

1. Do 5 reps and see how it feels. If it was easy, add 10 pounds to each side. If it was moderately hard, add 5 pounds to each side. If it was hard, add 2.5 pounds per side. Rest one minute then do another 5 reps.

2. Repeat this process until you can no longer do 5 reps.

3. At that point rest 10 minutes and attempt the last weight again. If you barely got it or failed on the last rep, use that as your 5 RM. If you got it and thought you could have pulled a few more, add 5 more pounds to the bar and try again. Repeat the process until you can't get 5 reps even after a 10-minute rest.

4. Once you've determined your 5 RM, multiply that number by 0.1 and add that to your 5 RM weight to calculate your 1 RM. So if your deadlift was 300 pounds, your 1 RM will be 300 + (300 x 0.1) or 330 pounds.

Whenever the workout calls for you to deadlift based on a percentage of your 1 RM, plug your number in and go. If the session calls for 5 sets of 10 deadlifts at 60 percent of your 1 RM, you'd multiply 330 by 0.6 and get 198 pounds as your working weight, then round that up to 200 since most places won't have 0.5- or 1-pound plates.

SUPPLEMENTAL EXERCISES

The following exercises will help you build greater endurance and strength, which will help you improve your deadlift.

Kettlebell Swings

The kettlebell swing is an awesome lift: It's dynamic, it raises the heart rate quickly and keeps it there, it builds strength and endurance of the hamstrings, glutes, lower back and core, and it teaches whole-body movement integration and acceleration and deceleration of an outside force. The idea behind the swing is simple. You dynamically load the posterior chain (hamstrings, glutes, lower back) by driving from the ground up, out through the legs, core, back and arms, and letting the momentum bring the arms and the kettlebell up in an arc from deep between your legs.

The movement is quite similar to the deadlift, but the main difference is that you don't drop the hips—they go straight back and the knees bend only enough to allow the hips to push back. The torso is in the same position as the start of the deadlift and ends with you standing and the arms at shoulder height.

Men should use at least a 16k (35 lb.) kettlebell, although 20 or 24k would be better. Start off with a moderate weight until you have the technique down. Women should be able to handle a 12k (26 lb.) kettlebell and be able to move the 16k bell after getting the movement down.

Performing the kettlebell swing several times per week in training will help create the strength-endurance your lower back needs to be able to pull 50 deadlifts at 135 pounds. Even if you can't get all 50 reps without a break, you should be able to break it up into sets that are manageable and don't put undue stress on your lower back.

Some Dos and Don'ts to remember when doing a kettlebell swing:

Do

- Keep the hips back, not down.
- Keep the back arched.
- Stay tight.
- Bend the knees slightly.
- Hike it between the legs.
- Drive through the mid-foot to the heel, and explode by bringing the hips forward and locking the knees.
- Keep the arms relaxed but not limp.
- Swing the bell no higher than the face.

Don't

- Don't round the lower back.
- Don't let the shins move.
- Don't lift the bell using the strength of the arms.
- Don't come up on the toes.
- Don't try to stop a swing on the upward phase.
- Don't try to stop a swing in the middle of the downward phase.

TWO-HAND KETTLEBELL SWING

1 Straddle the kettlebell, push your hips back, bend your knees and pick up the bell with both hands. Come to a standing position. (Note: Some instructors have you start with the bell on the floor. I've found that having beginners start from standing helps them learn the movement better.)

2–3 Push your hips back a little (don't let your hips go down, only back) then explode forward. Feel how the bell and your arms start to rock in unison with your hip movement. Don't try to forcibly move the bell with your arms; just let the momentum from your hips make it move. Each time, try to go a little farther back (think hiking a ball back between your legs), pushing your hips back more and exploding harder to bring the bell up higher; your forearms should touch your upper inner thigh at the end of the backswing. At the top, the bell should be nearly shoulder height— don't try to bring it overhead! The bell will feel like it's floating for a brief moment as the upward momentum stops and gravity kicks in; don't try to hold the bell up. At the apex, the bottom of the bell should be pointing in the same direction as your fist. Keep your wrist straight or the bell will flop around. Make sure your legs are doing the work. You shouldn't feel any undue stress in your shoulders or elbows; keep your shoulders

in their sockets by pinching your shoulder blades together and down. At this point, your entire body up to your chest should be tight. Your feet are locked, your hamstrings, glutes and quads are rigid, your hips are forward but not overextended. Your abs are braced like someone is about to punch you in the stomach.

To end the swing movement, simply lower your hips on the last reps and let the bell gently slide out of your hands; use your hamstrings and glutes to slow the bell. You can also just decrease the backward movement of your hips to slow down the movement, the opposite of the start of the swing.

DOUBLE BELL VARIATION: This can also be done holding a kettlebell in each hand. You'll need to widen your stance to make room for both kettlebells, but the mechanics are the same.

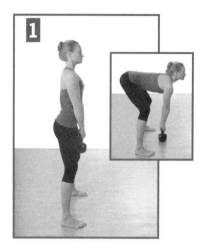

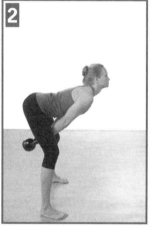

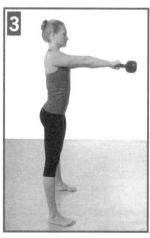

The one-hand swing is almost identical to the two-hand version; the main difference is that not as much power is transmitted to the arms into the bell so it won't move as high. Don't try to force it higher than it wants to go by lifting with your arms or bending backward.

1 Straddle the kettlebell, push your hips back, bend your knees and pick up the bell with one hand. Grip the bell toward the corner FARTHEST away from your lifting hand and use a thumb and forefinger grip. Come to a standing position but don't place your non-working hand on your thigh. Move it in unison with your working arm by placing it across the wrist of your working arm, or rest it on your hip or behind your back.

2 Keeping your chest square to the front, swing the kettlebell by driving your hips forward. It probably won't go as high as with the two-hand version—don't force it to.

3 When the bell hits its high point, it will hang briefly then start to fall. As it does so, bring your arm back between your legs at groin level while pushing your hips backward to avoid being hit by your forearm.

4 Snap your hips forward and let the bell come back up.

When you've finished your set, back off the power of the hip snap and reduce the depth of the backswing until you're barely rocking it, then set it on the floor. You can also lower your hips on the last set and let the bell come out of your hand and gently land on the ground. Once again, your legs do all the work.

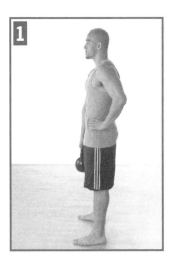

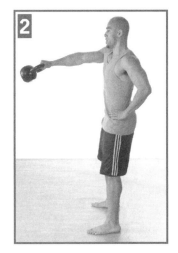

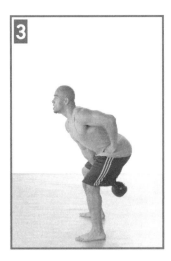

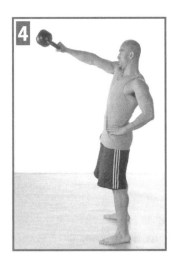

H2H KETTLEBELL SWING

1–3 Perform the One-Hand Kettlebell Swing (page 60). However, at the top of the swing, slip your other hand onto the handle while releasing with the first hand. Maintain the same structure as with a regular one-hand swing.

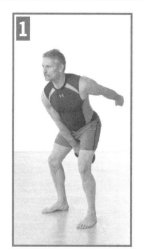
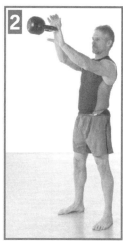
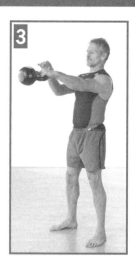

HIP EXTENSION

This is the same basic hip movement that you do during kettlebell swings. It helps open the hips, tone the glutes and stretch the hip flexors.

1 Lie on your back and bring your feet under your hips, keeping your heels down. Try to grab your ankles. If you can't reach them, use a towel, rope or yoga strap.

2 Squeeze your glutes and lift your hips as high as you can and pull on your ankles or the strap. Squeeze your knees as though you were trying to hold a small ball between them. Continue keeping your heels down.

Pause at the top, then lower your hips and repeat.

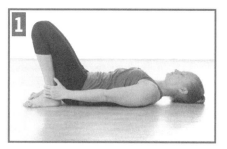
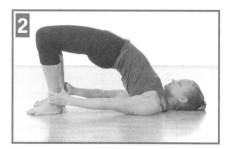

Kettlebell Deadlifts

The following deadlifts are all the same basic movement but with the weight in different places, which changes how the muscles are worked.

ONE-LEG DEADLIFT

1 Using a kettlebell or a dumbbell, stand with your feet together and the bell in your right hand. Shift your weight slightly to your right side, just enough to lift your left foot slightly off the floor.

2 Push your hips back and bend your right knee to let your hips go back and down. Keep your left leg straight behind you; your entire back from head to left foot should be one straight line and your hips should be lower than your shoulders. If you have the flexibility, try to place the kettlebell on the floor (you probably won't be able to do so with a dumbbell); don't tip over. Keep your abs tight to prevent hip rotation. Your chest should be out, your shoulders pulled back and, along with the hips, parallel to the floor.

3 Once you've gone down as far as you can without tilting over (don't let your hips get higher than your shoulders), drive through your heels, push your hips forward, straighten your right knee and stand up tall. You can set the left foot back down for balance if necessary at the top.

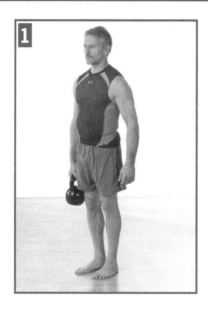

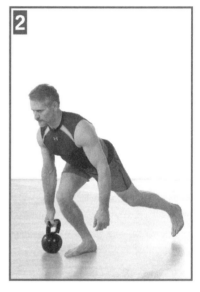

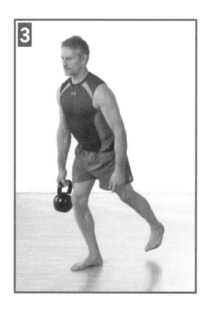

STIFF-LEGGED ONE-LEG DEADLIFT

1–2 Very similar to the One-Leg Deadlift (page 62), the stiff-legged version (where the standing leg isn't really stiff but bent slightly) uses the back more. You basically tilt at the hips to lift the bell. This is a great exercise for the lower back.

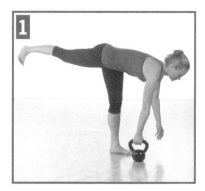
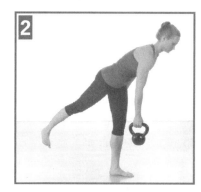

SUITCASE DEADLIFT

1 Stand with your knees and feet close but not quite together.

2 Keeping your chest up and your back arched, push your hips back as far as you can and bend your knees just a little to grab the handle of the kettlebell with your closest hand. Keep your arms soft but straight, just like with the kettlebell swing.

3 Drive your heels into the floor, push your hips forward and straighten your knees.

Push your hips back and bend your knees slightly to return the bell to the floor.

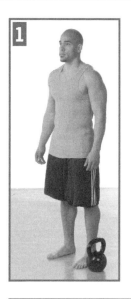
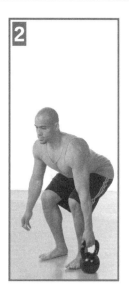
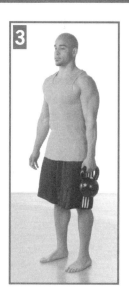

VARIATION: This can also be done with both hands. Using two bells works the core, especially the obliques, a bit differently than using one bell.

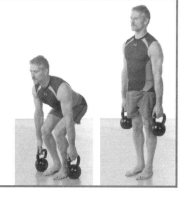

The sumo deadlift can be done with one or two kettlebells. In either case, you'll assume a wider-than-normal stance (feet at least shoulder-width apart), even wider if you're using two bells. The sumo deadlift works the inner thighs more than the suitcase deadlift.

1 Straddle the bell with a shoulder-width stance.

2 Push your hips way back, bend your knees a little, then grab the handle. Keep your chest lifted and your lower back arched.

3 Squeeze your abs, push your hips forward, straighten your knees and stand up tall with the bell between your legs; keep your hamstrings, glutes and abs tight.

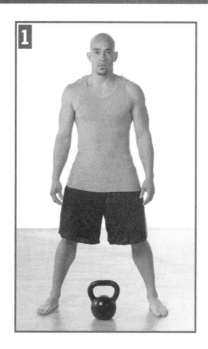

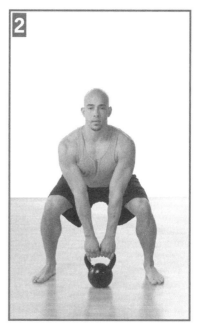

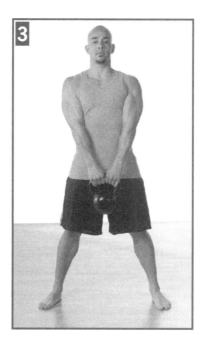

1–4

Using the steps described in the Sumo Deadlift (page 64), pick the bell up with one hand, locking your hips as you finish standing. This will make the bell almost float up. As your hips finish their extension, your arm and the bell will continue to rise slightly. At this point, switch hands quickly, push your hips back, touch the bell to the floor and keep going.

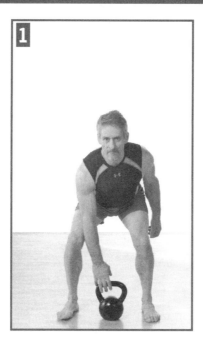

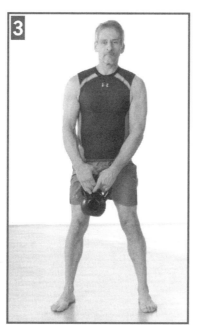

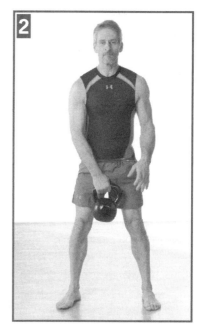

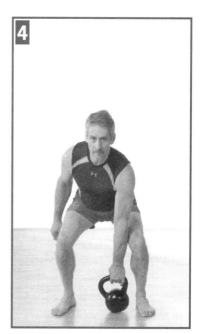

High Pulls

High pulls are a great conditioning movement that strengthens the upper back and shoulder complex, the abs and the posterior chain. There are several kettlebell movements that people call high pulls. This one (from Pavel Tsatsouline and Anthony Diluglio) focuses on scapular retraction and involves some coordination, timing and rhythm.

HIGH PULL

1 The high pull starts like a kettlebell swing. Start by doing several swings to refresh the movement.

2 As the bell reaches shoulder height, pull your shoulder blade back and let your elbow follow. As your shoulder retracts, your elbow should bend if your arm is soft; the bell should feel as if it's floating. Don't let the bell flop—the bottom should always point away, not up or down; make sure it stays in line with your wrist, which also should not bend up or down. Don't let your forearm go vertical; it should remain fairly close to parallel to the floor. Your elbow should wind up at about the height of your ear and almost straight to the side of your shoulder, staying just a little forward. It should also be a little higher than your shoulder.

3 Once your elbow has been pulled back, quickly and aggressively drive your arm out, allowing your elbow to straighten and your shoulder and shoulder blade to return to their normal position. Your arm should start to drop as it extends; at this point you're back in the regular swing descent.

Let the bell fall back between your upper thighs and explode back up and repeat. Maintain proper swing form throughout the upward and downward portions of the movement.

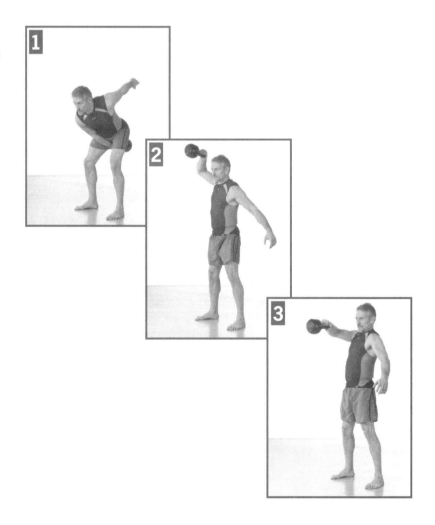

Push-ups

Push-ups. Everyone thinks they know how to do them, but I've seen countless pictures and videos on the Internet of people, including personal trainers, doing them wrong. I'll teach you how to do them correctly and I'll tell you why this is the correct way. Before long, you'll be doing 50 push-ups (or more) like a Spartan.

BODY POSITION

Varying the hand placement changes the muscles involved in a push-up. Bringing the hands together under the chest makes it a very triceps-intense exercise. Moving the hands wider than shoulder width puts most of the work in the chest. However, this wide hand position also places a lot of strain on the shoulders (the rotator cuff, for one) and can lead to injuries.

Placing the hands under the shoulders, or as close to under the shoulders as possible, is the correct hand placement for a push-up. Using this position will probably decrease your push-up numbers initially because the triceps are worked a lot harder than with the hands farther apart. But doing them this way will protect your shoulders and make your triceps insanely strong.

At the top position, the body alignment is exactly like you're standing tall with your arms out in front of you, shoulder high and slightly wider. The hips are locked in place (forward/down but not hyperextended) so you have a straight line from the back of your head to your feet. The feet should be between shoulder- and hip-width apart. (*Note:* Some trainers prefer an alternative position of keeping the back parallel to the floor at the top position.)

As the arms bend, the elbows should point backward, not out to the sides. The entire body stays locked in place, with the only movement coming from the bending arms. At the bottom position, the back is flat, parallel to the ground. The triceps and lats should be touching. The head should remain neutral, neither looking up nor tucking the chin under; the head should not move. I see many people who bob their heads when they do push-ups. This merely gives the exerciser the illusion that they're closer to the floor than they really are.

THE MOVEMENT

1 Start with your hands directly under your shoulders, or as close to that as you can get. Your arms should be straight but not locked out. Spread your fingers so that the middle fingers point straight ahead and the first and third finger point on the right hand to 11 and 1 and the reverse on the left; this helps spread the stress across the entire hand rather than put it in the wrist. Push the floor away so that your shoulder blades are not sticking out. You should be on the balls of your feet with your feet no more than shoulder-width apart. Keep your knees, glutes and abs locked tight. There should be a straight line from the base of your neck to your heels—do not lift your butt up or let it sag.

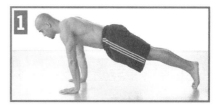

2 Slowly lower down, pointing your elbows to the rear, not to the sides. At the bottom position, your triceps and lats should touch.

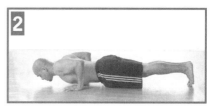

Return to the top position, making sure you're actively pushing the floor away.

DETERMINING YOUR CURRENT LEVEL

Now that you know how to do a proper push-up, let's see how many you can do. Do you do push-ups from your knees? Can you do any regular push-ups? If so, how many?

NUMBER OF PUSH-UPS	LEVEL
0–5	1 BEGINNER
5–10	2 INTERMEDIATE
10–15	3 INTERMEDIATE+
15+	4 ADVANCED

VARIATIONS & SUPPLEMENTAL EXERCISES

For beginners, we'll do static holds, short range of motion and some assistance work.

STATIC HOLD: TOP POSITION (HIGH PLANK)

1 Assume the top push-up position. Hold this position as long as you can:

    1 minute = poor
    2 minutes = fair
    3 minutes = good
    4 minutes = better
    5 minutes = excellent

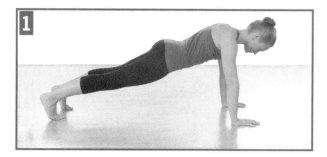

STATIC HOLD: MIDDLE POSITION

1 From top position, lower yourself halfway down and hold for as long as possible. Keep your elbows by your sides and your whole body tight.

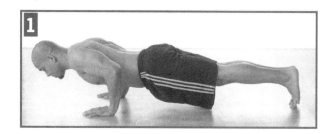

STATIC HOLD: BOTTOM POSITION (LOW PLANK)

The bottom hold is basically a plank on your hands instead of the forearms. When you can hold this and the top position for at least 3 minutes, you'll have developed some decent static core strength.

1 Lie on your stomach and place your hands under your shoulders. Your hands should be at your nipple line and in the same configuration as the high plank. Keeping your elbows by your sides and your whole body tight, press up just enough to roll onto the balls of your feet and lift the entire front of your body off the floor.

Don't raise your hips or let them sag or rotate. Your triceps and lats should be touching. Hold this for as long as possible.

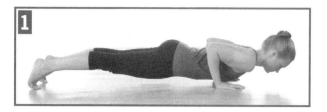

PARTIAL LOWER FROM HIGH PLANK

You only need to do 5 of these at a time as they're very demanding.

1–2 From the high plank, slowly lower yourself, leading with your chest, not your hips. Keep your elbows pointing toward the rear; don't let them flare out to the sides. Again, keep everything tight. When you can't go any lower without compromising your form, hold that position as long as you can then slowly raise back up.

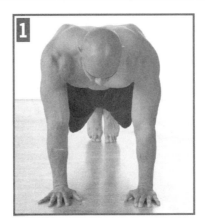
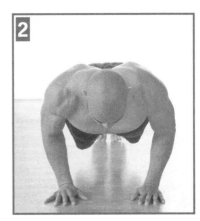

PARTIAL RAISE FROM LOW PLANK

1–2 From the low plank position, squeeze as hard as you can and try to lift yourself off the floor. The mistake most people make, and it's usually due to a weak core, is lifting the chest independently from the rest of the body. Keep everything rigid and the entire body moves as a unit. Go as high as you can, hold the position for as long as possible, and lower yourself slowly, maintaining proper form the entire time.

Over time you will be able to push up from plank and lower yourself from high plank and meet in the middle. At that point you should be able to do one correct push-up.

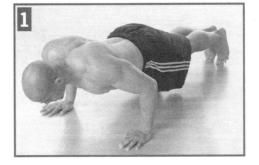
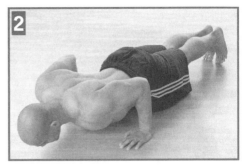

1 Place your right hand on a ball or kettlebell, your left hand on the floor. Your hands should be positioned as normal, except one is lifted.

2 Focusing on driving from the hand on the floor, perform a push-up.

3 Once you're in the high plank, move your left hand and your right foot at the same time so that your left hand is next to the kettlebell/ball.

4 Now take your right hand and your left foot and move them simultaneously so that your right hand is away from the bell and your feet are in proper push-up position.

5 Finally, pick up the hand closet to the bell and place it on the kettlebell and do another push-up. Keep going back and forth.

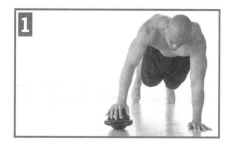

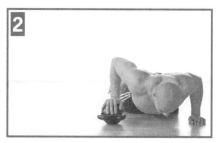

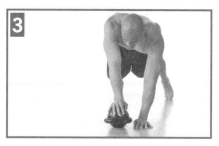

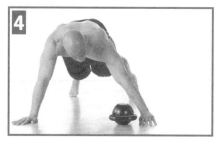

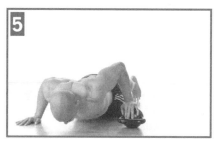

GETTING YOUR WEIGHT INTO POSITION

Once you have the weight(s) in hand, they should be held at chest level, the length of your forearm away from your body.

USING ONE DUMBBELL

1   Grab the center of the dumbbell from underneath, palm facing up.

2   Roll onto your side to face the weight; bring your other hand over and grab the weight, palm down.

3–4 Squeezing tightly, pin your elbow to the floor and roll back onto your back, using leverage to bring the bell to you.

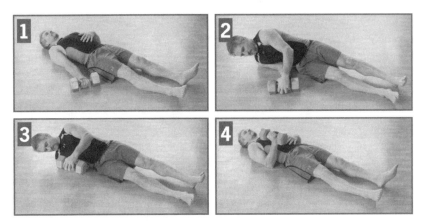

USING ONE KETTLEBELL

1   Hook your hand into the handle, palm face up, with the base of the hand under the little finger against the corner of the handle.

2   Roll onto your side to face the weight; bring your other hand over and grab the handle, palm down.

3   Squeezing tightly, pin your elbow to the floor and roll back onto your back, using leverage to bring the bell to you. At this point the arm holding the weight should be bent 90 degrees, with your forearm roughly level with the bottom of your ribs.

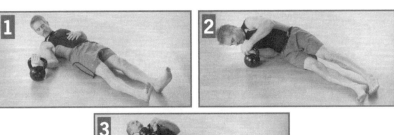

USING TWO DUMBBELLS

If you have a spotter, have them help you get the bells into place.

1 Once you have the first weight already in place as described on page 72, keep that arm tight against you and slip your other hand under the dumbbell, just like you did the first bell.

2 Roll to that side, using your elbow as a fulcrum; keep your other arm locked in place.

3 Keep both arms tight and roll flat onto your back. Remember to use leverage, not the strength of your shoulders or biceps, to bring the weight into position. Both arms should now be at your sides: elbows bent 90 degrees, forearms parallel to the floor, backs of the upper arms on the floor, palms facing each other.

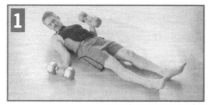
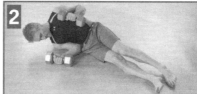
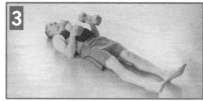

USING TWO KETTLEBELLS

1 Once you have the first bell already in place as described on page 72, take your other hand and position it in the kettlebell handle just as you did the first one, palm face up, bottom corner of the palm under the pinky in the far corner of the handle.

2 Stay tight and roll your body to the side of the arm you're using. Keep the first arm locked in place.

3 Squeezing tightly and keeping your arms locked against your body, roll flat onto your back. Remember to use leverage, not your muscles, to bring the bells up.

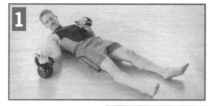
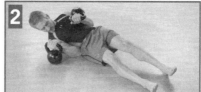
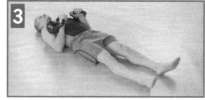

CHEST TOUCH

1 Start in a high plank position and lock everything tight, keeping your hips extended.

2 Quickly touch one hand to your chest and bring it back to the floor.

Repeat with the other arm. Move quickly but try to keep your hips from moving side to side or up and down.

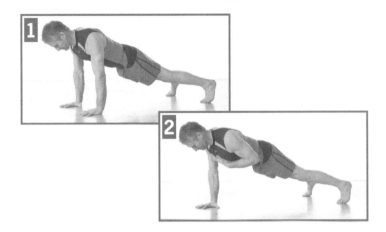

RENEGADE ROW

The pulling action of the row helps to offset the pushing movement of the push-up, maintaining or aiding the balance between the front and back of the upper body. You're also forced to support yourself on one arm, which will make your chest, triceps and abs stronger.

1–2 Assume a high plank and pull one hand back to your hip, utilizing your lats to retract your shoulder blade. Make sure you keep your hips and abs tight—there should be no rotation in the hips or waist.

Lower your hand and repeat on the other side.

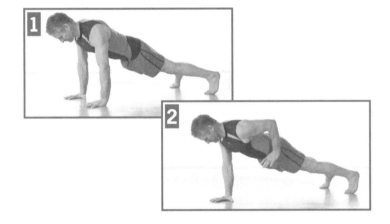

VARIATION: This can also be done with each hand on a kettlebell. Focus on driving the support hand through the bell and into the floor or the bell will tip over and you may get injured. Move slowly and with intent. Do not rush this movement. Squeeze the abs hard and pull the dumbbell or kettlebell to the hip. Slowly lower it, then repeat on the other side. Make sure you keep the hips and abs tight, with no rotation in the hips or waist.

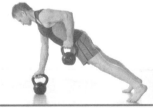

KETTLEBELL FLOOR PRESS

Being on the floor limits your range of motion, which will help keep your shoulders safe. You can do this same movement on a bench as well, but be careful not to go too low or you might strain or tear a pec or anterior deltoid.

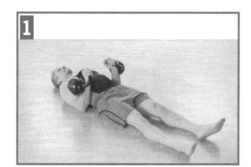

1 Lie on your back and get your kettlebells into position (pages 72–73). Keep your elbows bent 90 degrees, your triceps on the ground and your forearms perpendicular to the floor; the kettlebells should be on the back of your forearm, resting comfortably across your palm from the web of the thumb and forefinger to the base of your palm under your pinky at the wrist. Your palms can face either across your body (palms facing each other if you're using two weights) or toward your feet.

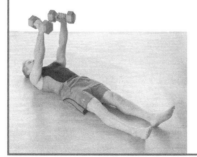

2 Squeeze everything (abs, glutes, quads, toes) and press the weight up, focusing on your lats. Lock out your elbows. Your hands should not travel toward your head; they should still be in line with your chest or slightly below.

To bring the bells down, PULL them as though someone were holding them, preventing you from getting them back down. This will work the eccentric or negative portion of the movement and is similar to doing a slow descent during the push-up. You should really feel the lats working during this part of the movement.

VARIATION: This can also be done with dumbbells.

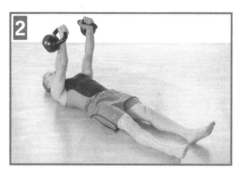

SINGLE KETTLEBELL FLOOR PRESS VARIATION: With both bells locked out, pull one down and press it back up repeatedly for the allotted time interval. Then switch sides. This is one set.

STATIC HOLD VARIATION: Keep both bells locked out over your chest.

This is a different movement than when done with a dumbbell and a bench. Throughout the movement, keep the arm close to the body and focus on using the lat and shoulder blade, not the shoulder; in addition, prevent any movement other than the arm and shoulder complex—the torso does not rotate or move up and down, and the hips and shoulder girdle stay locked in place. You should feel your obliques working hard to prevent this movement.

1 Step one leg forward and the other leg back, bending your front knee and keeping your back knee straight but not hyperextended; your front shin should be perpendicular to the floor and your back foot should be turned out at a comfortable angle (but not more than 45 degrees). Keep your back foot between two parallel lines, one from the hip and the other from the shoulder. Place the kettlebell on the floor by the big toe of your front foot; the handle should be parallel to your foot. Place your forearm across your front thigh, just above your knee. (If your left foot is forward, your left arm is across your thigh.) Try to keep your shoulders and hips parallel to the floor.

2 Grab the kettlebell by the front corner of the handle and tilt the bell back toward your hip; bring your elbow back at an angle so that the kettlebell moves toward the outside of your hip (think about putting your hand in your pants pocket). Keep your back flat, your abs tight, and your chest up, and pinch your shoulder blades together.

Continue to stay tight and lower the kettlebell back to the floor by the front foot.

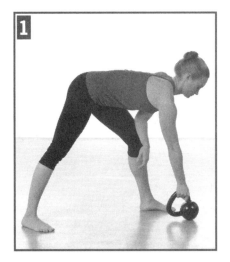

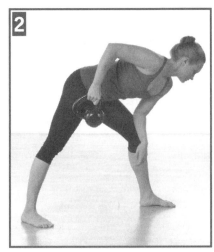

DECLINE PUSH-UP

This variation places more of your body weight onto your hands, arms, shoulders and chest.

1–2 Place your feet on a sturdy box, bench or chair and your hands on the floor. Perform a proper push-up as usual, but be especially careful to not let your hips sag; you should still lead with your chest.

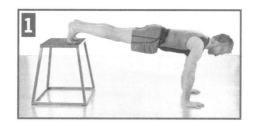

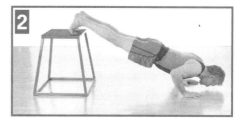

TRIANGLE PUSH-UP

You should feel this push-up mostly in the triceps.

1 Position your hands together under your sternum, forming a triangle with the first finger and thumb of both hands.

2 Lower yourself as far as you can without losing form, then drive back up.

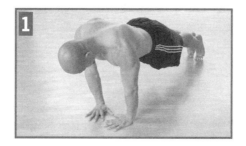

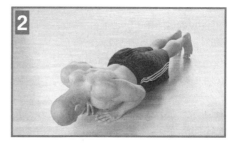

INCLINE PUSH-UP

You'll have to experiment a bit to find the right height for this push-up. You want it to be hard to do a full push-up, but not so hard you can't do at least 5. If you can do 10 or more easily, lower the platform.

1 Place your hands on a sturdy box, bench or chair—just make sure it can't slide. Keep your feet on the floor and maintain the same alignment as in a regular push-up.

2 Lower yourself down, then drive back up.

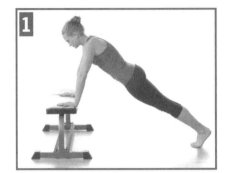

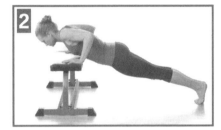

WIDE PUSH-UP

These push-ups are used to hit the pecs harder, but they should be practiced sparingly due to the stress they place on the shoulder.

1–2 Perform the push-up with your hands wider than shoulder-width apart. Your hands should still be in line with your shoulders, not out in front of you. The depth of this push-up will be slightly less than the regular push-up; don't go too low as you may stress your rotator cuff.

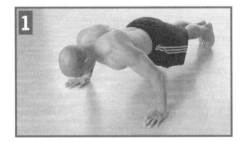

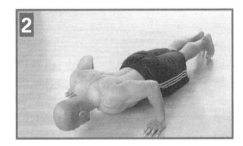

Box Jumps

Box jumps sound and look easy, but they're deceptively hard, especially if you're jumping to a 24-inch box, as suggested in the Spartan Warrior Workout. For many people, the box jump requires a "leap of faith." Common subconscious fears include jumping up and banging the shins, doing a face plant on the box or missing the box entirely. Luckily, the box height is scalable, and if you harbor any of these trepidations, use a lower box until the fear goes away and your legs get stronger.

Since the workout calls for 50 box jumps, don't push too hard too soon or you may find yourself face first on the box.

BODY POSITION

Jumping, when not done properly, can be hard on the joints. In order to prevent injury when doing box jumps, there are several things you need to keep in mind. Pay close attention to your knees when you're on the ground and when you land on top of the box. Make sure they track with the feet (i.e., knees point in the same direction as the toes); don't let them collapse inward. Also, don't land stiff legged—always land on the balls of your feet while sinking your hips back and down, loading the legs to prepare for the next jump.

EQUIPMENT

The Spartan Warrior Workout calls for a 24-inch box. You can purchase one from many online vendors; those are typically metal but, searching the Internet, you should be able to find a blueprint detailing how to make your own out of wood. If you're short, you'll have a much tougher time jumping to a 24-inch box than someone with long legs. If 24 inches is too high, drop to 20; try not to go lower than 18 inches, though. A good rule of thumb is the top of the box should hit about mid-thigh. Ladies, your minimum box height is 12 inches but you should try for 18.

THE RIGHT HEIGHT

One way to tell if you can jump onto a box of a certain height is to do a jump tuck. You'll need a witness and a box.

Stand next to the box, bend your knees and jump as high as you can, tucking your knees to your chest.

Your witness should determine if your feet come up higher than the box and, if so, how much higher. If you have a few inches of clearance, you can jump onto that box.

We normally advocate barefoot training whenever possible, but for box jumps we wear shoes to protect the balls of the feet. Jumping places a tremendous amount of stress on the feet and jumping up onto a wooden or metal surface will eventually cause injury to the feet. The shoes should provide some padding but need to be flat and firm, *not* a running shoe or cross-trainer. Appropriate footwear would be a hiking shoe or something like the old Chuck Taylor Converse high or low tops.

Running shoes or cross-trainers are designed to absorb the force from running. However, when lifting weights (whether doing deadlifts or kettlebell swings), the last thing you want is for the shoes to absorb the power you're trying to generate. In addition, running shoes and cross-trainers are notoriously unstable and can cause many problems with the ankles turning over. This instability can cause the knees to collapse when squatting or deadlifting and tend to make you shift your weight to your toes on movements like the kettlebell swing. My clients normally train barefoot and many people question that, usually asking what happens if they drop the weight. My answer (from Jeff Martone) is that "fast feet are happy feet." You'll automatically get your feet out of the way if you drop the weight. But unless you're wearing solid-steel shoes, you're going to have a broken foot no matter what type of footwear you choose.

However, because we're doing box jumps, we need to wear shoes that will protect the feet. "Chucks" work just fine, especially since we don't want to take time to put shoes on in the middle of the workout.

THE MOVEMENT

1 Stand with your feet comfortably apart, hip to shoulder width.

2 Push your hips back and down into a quarter squat. Your torso should be angled and your arms should reach back at the same angle as your back.

3–4 Explode forward—not straight up—so that you land on the box. Use your arms to generate momentum by raising them up in front of you as you jump. At the same time, bring your knees up just enough to clear the box. Land with the balls of your feet touching the box first, then your heels. Try to land softly, like a cat, making little to no noise. Once you've landed, stand up, bringing your hips through. Don't stop short. Many people who do box jumps don't extend their hips and therefore miss getting the full benefits of this very powerful movement. The reason they fail do to this is because it's harder and takes longer; it's considered cheating if you don't stand tall at the top.

To return to the floor, push your hips back and down slightly and drive back with the balls of your feet. Don't try to straighten out your legs; they should be slightly bent and ready to absorb the force of the body landing on the floor. Be light and sink your hips as your feet hit the floor. You should be in the start position. As soon as you land, explode back up and repeat. Avoid letting your heels touch the ground when you land as this will dissipate the energy stored in your legs and will take you longer to execute the next jump.

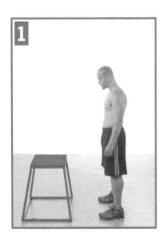 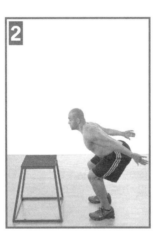 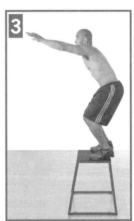 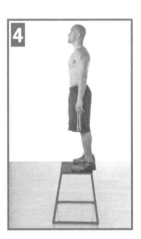

VARIATIONS & SUPPLEMENTAL EXERCISES

These assistance exercises will help not only the box jump but will also give you more overall explosive power. You should see an improvement in your regular squats, both front and back, and if you play a sport that involves jumping, you should see massive gains in your jump height and endurance.

Jump squats should first be performed with body weight alone. Later, you may be ready to add extra weight. In learning to jump you must also learn to land. Improper landing technique will jar the body and can wreck your knees and lower back. To start, we'll do jumps without leaving the ground to practice the landing.

1–2 Stand with your feet about shoulder-width apart and pointed forward or turned out slightly. Staying flat-footed, pull yourself down as deep as you can go without leaning forward. Push your arms down hard behind you to give you extra power.

3 Explode upward but keep your toes on the floor as your hips fully extend (note: photo shows full squat jump). Once fully extended, sink your hips back and down, letting your knees bend, and sink back onto your heels or as deep as you can go, the same as the initial squat in steps 1–2. Be graceful and soft—no jarring of the body.

Once you've mastered that, you can jump off the floor, keeping your legs fairly straight and your feet just a few inches off the floor. Use the same soft landing. Make contact with the balls of your feet first, then sink back onto your heels as your hips sink down, dropping back into a deep squat; repeat without pausing.

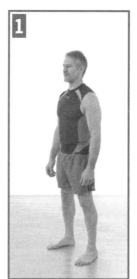
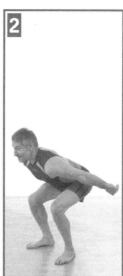
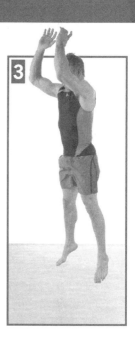

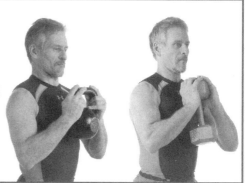

VARIATION: Holding the kettlebell or dumbbell in your hands, drop into a quarter squat and jump as high as you can. Land softly, sink back into the quarter squat and repeat.

The jump tuck is very explosive since you have to violently pull both knees up as high as possible without the benefit of squatting to use the hamstrings and glutes.

1 Stand with your feet about shoulder-width apart and pointed forward or turned out slightly.

2 Contracting your hip flexors powerfully, bring your knees to your chest as quickly as possible, keeping your torso erect.

Land by quickly extending your hips and knees as you return to the ground. As soon as the balls of your feet touch the floor, pull your knees back up to your chest—don't allow your heels to contact the floor.

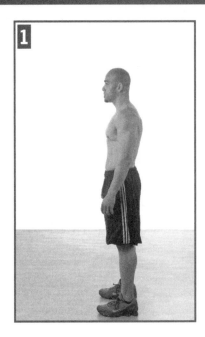

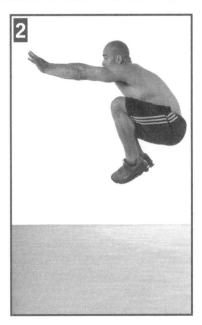

MODIFICATION: If you have trouble with this, practice the double mountain climber. This is the same explosive contraction of the hip flexors you do when performing the standing jump tuck, but being in a push-up position makes it a little easier to do and allows you to practice the movement without worrying so much about the coordination and timing. You may find your abs sore the next day.

1 Start in a high plank position.

2 Without raising your hips, bring both knees to your chest at the same time as quickly as possible, your feet coming under you.

3 As soon as your toes touch the floor, drive your legs back to the high plank position and repeat.

STATIC LUNGE

1 Step one foot out a little farther than your natural step.

2 Bend knees until they're 90 degrees and your front thigh is parallel with the floor. Your back heel should be lifted almost 90 degrees throughout the movement. Keep your torso upright.

3 Drive off your front foot, keeping your heel down; your back foot should only help you maintain your balance. As soon as both knees are straight, sink back down until you're in a deep lunge.

Switch sides.

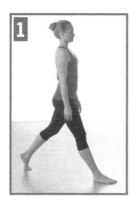
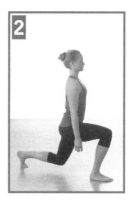
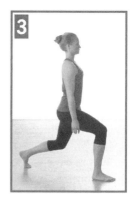

When performing the static lunge, there is no forward/backward movement of the hips. The hips travel on a straight line up and down.

FORWARD/BACKWARD LUNGE

1 Stand with your feet hip-width apart.

2 Leading with the heel, step forward with your right foot. The distance should be a little more than your normal stride length and your feet should remain in line with the hips. Sink your hips straight down while simultaneously bending both knees approximately 90 degrees; keep your torso vertical at all times and your abs and glutes tight. Your front shin should be vertical and your weight should be on the mid- to back part of your front foot; the heel of your back foot should be almost vertical. Keep your hips parallel to the floor. Point both feet and knees straight ahead at all times.

Push back off the mid-portion of your front foot and stand up. At this point you can either step forward with the same foot or the other.

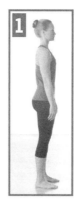
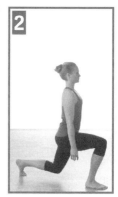

BACKWARD VARIATION: From standing, step straight back so that the ball of your foot is on the floor and your heel is up. Your feet should still be hip-width apart. Once your foot makes contact with the floor, sink your hips straight down. Your position should be exactly the same as the forward lunge.

Sometimes called Bulgarian split squat, this works the glutes, quads and hamstrings while decreasing pressure on the spine. Your best bet is to use a bench press bench, although a flat, preferably padded, surface about 19 to 20 inches high works well, too. If the stretch to the elevated quadriceps is too much or you're short, use a shorter platform. You may want to place a small pad under the rear knee to keep it from banging on the floor.

1 Place the top of one foot on the bench, pointing the knee down; your other foot should be forward enough so that your shin is vertical when your front thigh is parallel to the floor. Straighten your front leg. Keep your torso upright throughout the exercise.

2 Bend both knees to lower your hips until your front thigh is parallel to the floor. If you feel excessive stretching through the hip flexor and quadriceps of the elevated leg, you need to stretch more; in the meantime don't go quite so deep.

Return to standing by driving with the front foot. Minimize the use of the elevated foot. It's on the bench for balance, not to help you move or stand. Keep your front foot flat on the floor throughout the entire movement.

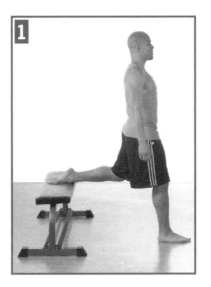

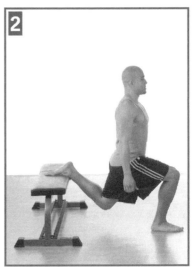

VARIATION: Once you can do the unloaded movement properly, you can challenge yourself by holding a kettlebell or dumbbell chest high with both hands (the goblet position) or holding one in each hand with your arms along your sides.

1–3 Stand in front of a sturdy box or other platform and step up onto it. Try to lift your knee and foot straight up. If you notice your foot moving to the outside or inside to clear the box, you'll need to work on your hip flexibility (see pages 131–32 for some appropriate stretches).

Step back with the same foot you started with.

VARIATION: You can also add a backward lunge when you step back by planting the foot firmly on the floor. Instead of bringing the other foot down next to the first (which would bring you to standing), move that foot behind you just as in the Backward Lunge (page 83).

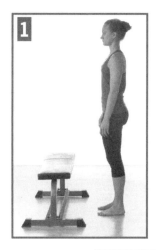

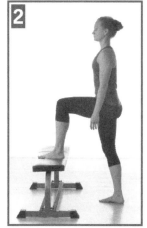

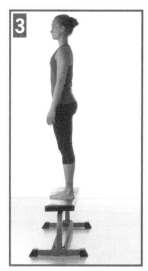

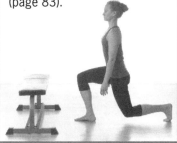

JUMPING LUNGE

These are very advanced so don't try these until you're comfortable with regular lunges.

1-3 Start in a lunge position and explode upward. Keep your arms relaxed, elbows bent and hands about chest high. As you reach your peak, switch legs and land in a lunge. As the balls of your feet contact the floor, bend your knees so you sink straight down. As with all lunge variations, your bottom position is the same as in the forward, backward and static lunges. Don't let your back knee slam into the ground.

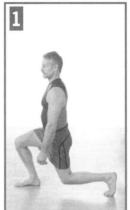
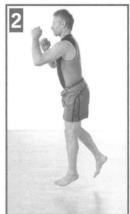
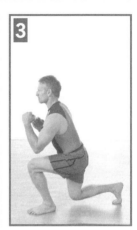

DEPTH JUMP

This is a true plyometric exercise and should be done early in your workout—and only for a short interval or a few reps; they're very demanding.

1-4 Stand on a box, fall off (as opposed to stepping off) and explode back up, jumping as high as you can or onto another box.

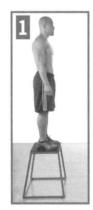
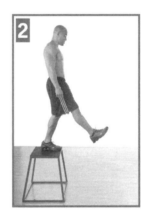
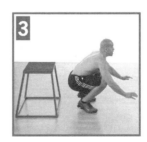
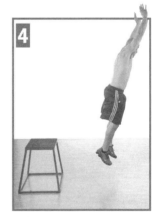

Floor Wipers

The Spartan Warrior Workout calls for 50 floor wipers. These are an interesting and demanding exercise in which you lie flat on your back while holding a barbell locked out, touch your feet to the plates on one side of the bar, lower them without touching the floor, then bring them up to touch the plates on the other side of the bar. Essentially you're doing a static chest press hold and rotational legs raises. All this involves upper body strength and stability as well as extreme core strength and flexibility. You'll want a spotter to help you with the barbell.

BODY POSITION

Your grip on the bar should be slightly wider than your shoulders, almost where they would be if you were doing a push-up. Keep your thumb wrapped around the bar for safety. Make sure your spotter is paying attention! When your legs are straight out in front of you, keep your lower back pressed into the floor at all times. If you find yourself arching your lower back when lowering your legs, bend your knees slightly to avoid straining it.

EQUIPMENT

You'll need a barbell and up to 135 pounds of weight—which is what the workout calls for. If you've done a lot of bench pressing, you shouldn't have a problem with 135; otherwise, drop down to a more suitable poundage. Inexperienced guys should try it with 95 pounds to start and see how it feels. Women should start off with an empty bar and work up from there.

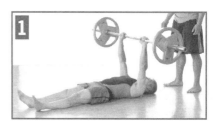

Also, just in case, you'll need a spotter—someone who can lift and hold the weight you'll be working with. If you prefer to use a squat rack, make sure the pins or hooks are set so they're high enough to keep the bar off your chest when you're resting under it. No cracked ribs or broken faces, please!

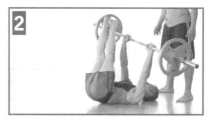

THE MOVEMENT

1 Lie flat on the floor, legs straight, and press the barbell above your chest, locking out your arms. Keep everything tight.

2 Keeping your legs straight and feet together throughout the movement, lift your feet up and touch the plates on one side of the bar.

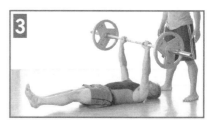

3–4 Lower your feet toward the floor but don't touch it. Be careful to press your lower back into the floor so you don't arch it, which will lead to an injury. Now raise your feet to touch the plates on the other side of the bar. That's one rep.

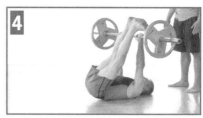

DETERMINING YOUR CURRENT LEVEL

As mentioned earlier, if you've been weightlifting for more than three months or so, you should be able to handle 135 pounds easily in a lock-out position; women, you should be able to handle 95 pounds.

If you're unsure, use a squat rack with the safety bars set to just below your arm extension and load the bar with the prescribed weight. If you can push it up those last few inches without excessive strain or arching your back, hold it there as long as you can, keeping track of the time. If you can't hold the lock-out, drop down 10 pounds and try again.

Keep dropping weight until you find a weight that is easy to lock-out and that you can hold for at least 30 seconds. This will be your working weight for the floor press.

While holding the bar locked out, try the leg movement a few times to see how it feels. You should be able to get a few reps (remember, you have to touch the plates on each side of the bar once to equal one rep).

ASSISTANCE EXERCISES

In the beginning stages you should practice the ab work (leg movement) separately from the barbell static hold. This will allow you to focus on getting stronger in each component. Once you get the hang of the leg movement and have built up some endurance in the static hold, you can combine the two.

STATIC HOLD

For beginners, the static hold will probably be harder than the leg raises. Have your spotter help you get the bar up and to be ready to take it if you can't hold it, or use the safety bars on a squat rack and load the bar onto them.

1 Once you're under the bar with your hands properly positioned, squeeze everything

and drive the bar up, locking your elbows and keeping them locked. Hold the bar as long as you can then put it back on the pins/hooks or have your spotter take the bar and put it back on the rack. Practice holding the bar for 3-minute sets. At first you'll probably struggle with 1-minute sets, but you must persevere.

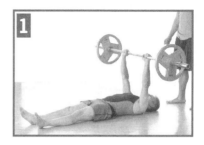

VARIATION: This can also be done with kettlebells or dumbbells.

Assistance Exercises for the Static Hold

BENCH PRESS

Unlike the floor wiper, you perform the bench press while lying on a bench. This allows fuller range of motion but also adds difficulty because moving the bar off your chest the first few inches is the toughest part.

1 Have your spotter help you lower the bar to your chest. Keep your hands a little wider than shoulder-width apart and your feet flat on the floor. If you can't reach the floor, stack some plates until your feet are flat on them.

2 Squeeze the bar. Focus on pressing from your lats (armpit muscles), not from your chest and shoulders, and straighten your elbows. Pause at the top and slowly bring the bar back to your chest. Work the negative eccentric portion hard. It'll make you sore but will also crank up your strength quickly.

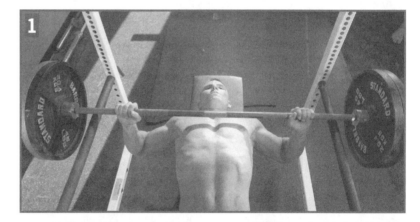

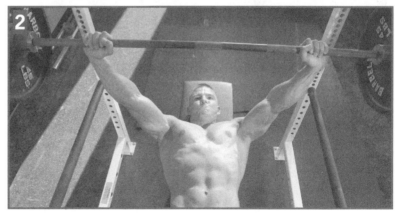

DETERMINING YOUR BENCH PRESS 1 REP MAX (RM)

Use the table below to figure your starting weight. Have a spotter ready or use a squat rack with the safety bars set so that the bar almost touches your chest.

EXPERIENCE LEVEL	WOMEN	MEN
Never benched	45 lb. (empty bar)	95 lb.
Benched a few times	65 lb.	115 lb.
Benched consistently for a few months	95 lb. or last session weight	135 lb. or last session weight
Benched consistently for a year-plus	your last session weight	your last session weight

1   Attempt to press the weight 5 times. If it was easy, add 10 pounds (two 5-pound plates) to the bar and do another rep. If it was hard, add 5 pounds (two 2.5-pound plates) and try again.

2   Keep adding weight until you can no longer get 5 reps. Rest 10 minutes and try the same weight. If you got it and you feel as though you could've gotten another rep, load 5 more pounds, rest 5 minutes and give it a go. If you barely got 5 or failed after your minute rest, you have your 5 RM weight. If you added to the bar after adding 5 pounds and resting 5 minutes, you should be pretty close to your max. This is rather subjective but you'll be close enough.

Once you have your 5 RM number, multiply it by 0.1 to determine your 1 RM. For example, if your 5 RM was 200, multiply it by 0.1 (20 pounds) and add that to your 5 RM weight. In this case your 1 RM would end up being 220 pounds (200 + [200 x 0.1]). Use that number whenever a percentage of 1 RM is called for in the workout.

Assistance Exercises for the Static Hold

PUSH-UP

See the push-up section on page 67 for full details on how to do various kinds of push-ups. The more you do the stronger you'll be, but body weight alone will only get you so far. If you're already comfortable with push-ups, you may want to add a weight vest or have your training partner place his hands on your shoulders to apply some resistance. Another way to add extra weight is to have your partner place a weight plate across your upper back. Just be careful and don't overdo it. Also continue to maintain strict form—adding additional weight to bodyweight exercises can make you get sloppy. Remember: Don't go to failure. Keep your form clean and solid.

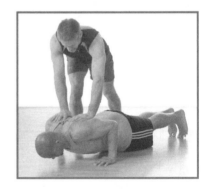

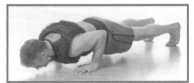

KETTLEBELL FLOOR PRESS

Being on the floor limits your range of motion, which will help keep your shoulders safe. You can do this same movement on a bench as well, but be careful not to go too low or you might strain or tear a pec or anterior deltoid.

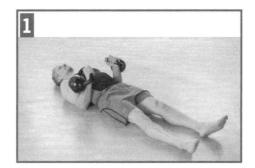

1 Lie on your back and get your kettlebells into position (pages 72–73). Keep your elbows bent 90 degrees, your triceps on the ground and your forearms perpendicular to the floor; the kettlebells should be on the back of your forearm, resting comfortably across your palm from the web of the thumb and forefinger to the base of your palm under your pinky at the wrist. Your palms can face either across your body (palms facing each other if you're using two weights) or toward your feet.

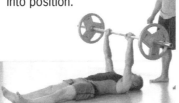

2 Squeeze everything (abs, glutes, quads, toes) and press the weight up, focusing on your lats. Lock out your elbows. Your hands should not travel toward your head; they should still be in line with your chest or slightly below.

To bring the bells down, PULL them as though someone were holding them, preventing you from getting them back down. This will work the eccentric or negative portion of the movement and is similar to doing a slow descent during the push-up. You should really feel the lats working during this part of the movement.

VARIATION: This can also be done with a barbell or dumbbells. See pages 72–73 on how to get your dumbbell into position.

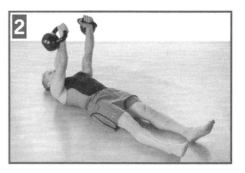

SINGLE KETTLEBELL FLOOR PRESS VARIATION: With both bells locked out, pull one down and press it back up repeatedly for the allotted time interval. Then switch sides. This is one set.

STATIC HOLD VARIATION: Keep both bells locked out over your chest.

LEG RAISE

1 Lie flat on the floor with your arms out to the sides at shoulder height, palms down. Try to keep your back flat on the floor at all times.

2 Keeping your legs straight, raise your feet up to one side. Press your hands into the floor to keep you from falling to the side.

3 Lower them back to the floor (but don't touch!) and raise them up to the other side. At no point will you be raising your legs straight up the middle; do not rotate your hips from side to side.

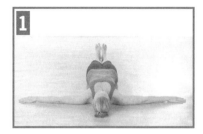

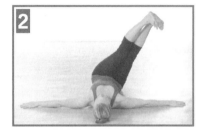

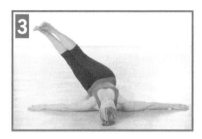

Assistance Exercises for the Leg Raise

LEG THRUST

If you experience lower back discomfort, place your hands under your hips. This exercise really hits the entire rectus abdominis, from the diaphragm to the pelvis.

1 Lie on your back with your legs straight, then lift your feet until your hips are at a 90-degree angle to your waist; keep your feet straight over your hips. You can place your hands behind your head or by your sides.

2 Now point your toes and drive your hips up as high as you can, keeping your legs perpendicular to the floor. Your weight is on your upper back and shoulders, not your neck.

3 Lower your hips back down, then, still keeping your knees straight, lower your feet to the floor until they're about 2 inches off the floor.

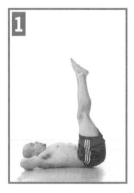

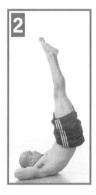

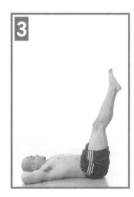

PLANK

The standard plank is another core exercise focusing on stability.

1 Place your forearms on the floor parallel to each other; align your elbows under your shoulders. You may keep your palms face down on the floor or make fists and place the meaty part of the fist on the floor. Extend your legs behind you like you would when doing a push-up, keeping your hips in the same plane as your shoulders. Squeeze your abs, glutes, hamstrings, quads, arms—everything but your neck— and hold that position. Make sure your back is flat and that your hips are level with your shoulders; don't let your back sag or your hips go high or low. Maintain this position for as long as you can, the longer the better:

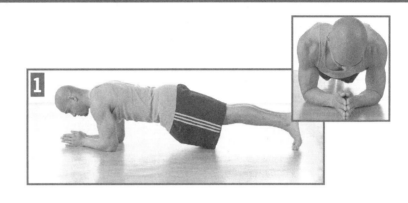

    1 minute = poor
    2 minutes = fair
    3 minutes = good
    4 minutes = better
    5 minutes = excellent

HIGH PLANK

Assume the top position of a push-up, placing your hands on the floor in line with your shoulders, keeping your back flat, your knees straight and your hips in the same plane as your shoulders. Squeeze everything and hold it for as long as you can.

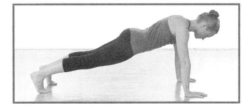

BIRD DOG

START POSITION: Start with your hands under your shoulders and both knees on the floor, under your hips. Two basic phases precede the full bird dog—once you can hold either arm out for at least 30 seconds and you can do the same with each leg with no rotation, it's time to do the full bird dog.

1 In the most basic version, lift one arm straight out in front of you at shoulder height, fingers pointing straight ahead, and hold it. Don't let your hips rotate; they and your shoulders should remain parallel to the floor. If you can hold this easily for at least 30 seconds on each side, move on to the next level.

2 For the next phase, keep both hands on the floor and lift one leg off the floor so that the leg is level with the hip and the toes point straight back. Stay tight and don't let your torso rotate. Your hips should remain parallel to the floor.

3 For the full bird dog, lift one leg and the opposite arm. As with the easier progressions, your hips and shoulders should remain parallel to the floor. There should be a straight line from your heel to your fingers. Remember: You're going across the body, right foot and left hand and vice versa.

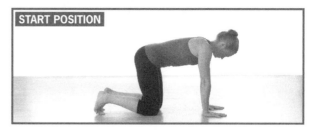

START POSITION

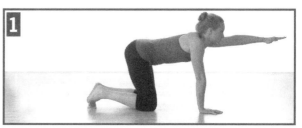

1

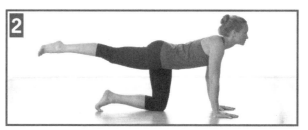

2

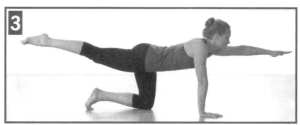

3

PLANK VARIATION: If you can do the full bird dog for at least one minute per side, try the full bird dog from a high plank position. This is very tough.

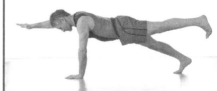

RENEGADE ROW

Done correctly, these are as much about using the abs to prevent rotation as they are about working the lats. You'll need two hex dumbbells or two kettlebells.

1 Place your bells under your shoulders so that your palms face each other (the handles should run parallel to your body). Take a high plank position and spread your feet a little farther apart than you would for push-ups. Your foot position can make these easier or harder; the closer together they are, the harder they are because your base of support is narrower, which makes your obliques work harder to stabilize you.

2 Now stay tight and drive your energy down into the floor like the bells aren't there. Squeeze and pull one bell to your hip; it will move at an angle. Don't let your hips rotate; you should feel your obliques a lot.

Slowly lower the bell to the floor. Once it's there, shift your energy to that side, drive into the ground and pull the other bell to your hip. Alternate sides rather than do all the reps on one side then the other. Switching sides forces the abs to work hard because the stabilizers have to keep moving based on the shifting of the stress.

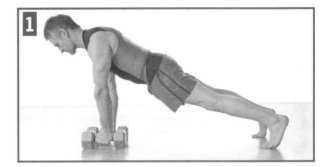

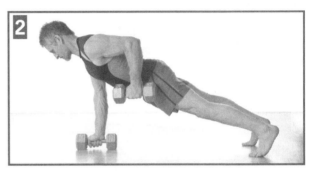

VARIATION: An easier version is to use no weight and to bring your hand to touch your chest before placing it back on the ground. These are especially hard if you go very slowly, using a 5 count up, a 5 count hold and a 5 count lower.

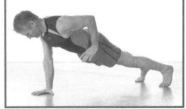

RUSSIAN TWIST

1 Sit on the ground with your feet off the floor. Hold a kettlebell or dumbbell high in front of your chest, keeping your elbows in and down.

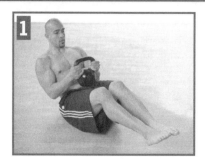

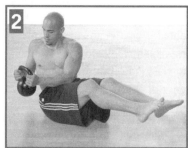

2–3 Rotate from side to side about 20 degrees from center, letting your head follow the bell. If you have lower back problems or find this uncomfortable (not just hard), then keep your feet on the floor with your knees bent.

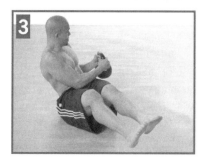

VARIATION: This can also be done with a medicine ball.

UNICYCLE

1 Lie flat on your back and place your left hand behind your head. Lift both feet about 6 inches off the floor.

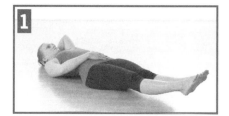

2 Contract your abs and bring your lift elbow toward your hips and your right knee toward your elbow. They should meet halfway. The other leg should remain extended and about 6 inches off the floor. Don't pull on your neck with your hand!

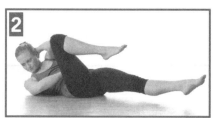

Extend your left leg and lower your torso so you're flat again.

After performing a set, switch sides, right elbow and left knee. You'll feel this in your obliques while doing them but probably around your diaphragm the next day.

Dead Clean and Press

The dead clean and press (DCP) is considered a combination movement and is one of the principle movements used by kettlebell lifters. The dead clean helps build explosive strength, speed and timing while the press teaches total body tension, using the whole body to move the weight, and promotes shoulder health.

The clean is a very powerful movement, especially when initiated from the floor, or "dead" position. It's "dead" because you're moving a dead weight as opposed to using a pendulum motion to bring the bell to rack. The force necessary to lift the bell comes from the ground up and is generated by squatting down, exploding upward and using momentum to sneak the hand through the handle so the bell lands softly against the back of the forearm.

For the Spartan Warrior Workout, you'll need to do 25 on each side for a total of 50.

BODY POSITION

There are many technical details in learning to clean properly, but the main points are to use the legs, not the back; to keep a relaxed grip; and to let the bell rotate around the hand, not over the fist. Done correctly, it's a very fluid movement with no impact to the forearm. If it bangs you, you aren't doing it correctly!

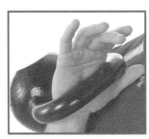
Correct way to grab the bell

There are a few points to be aware of: First and foremost, this is NOT a curl. You should NOT feel this in the biceps. As the bell comes up, try to keep the thumb side of the hand in toward the body—that is, don't turn the palm out or up. There should be no banging of the forearm. If you're banging, you're probably letting the bell come over the fist or squeezing the handle too hard. Shove the hand through the handle; this will make the bell wrap around the forearm rather than over the fist and makes for a much smoother, more fluid movement.

In the "rack" position, the hand should be at or below the level of the collar bone; the forearm should be vertical or tilted in toward the body. The corner of the kettlebell handle rests against the bone on the outside edge of the heel of the hand, same as for the floor press. Some refer to this as the "hip of the hand."

THE MOVEMENT

1 Begin with the bell on the floor between your feet and slightly behind you. Turn the bell so the handle is 45 degrees back toward the side opposite of the hand you're going to use. If you're using your right hand, turn the handle toward your left rear. Grab the bell with your thumb and forefinger near the back corner of the handle; wrap your other fingers around, but your thumb and forefinger will be doing most of the work. Keep your grip relaxed, just tight enough to hold the bell. Bend your knees and sink your hips down into a partial squat; your arm should be straight with no slack in it.

2–3 Now explode straight up and, bringing your hips forward, think about doing a vertical jump. The bell will come up as your torso does. At that point, drop your elbow into your lower ribs and shoot your hand through the handle. The bell should wrap around your fist and lie against your forearm. You should be in the "rack" position as described in "Body Position" above, with your elbow in against your lower ribs, your palm facing about 45 degrees inward toward your body and your forearm fairly vertical.

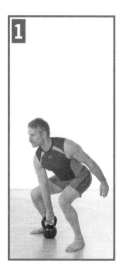 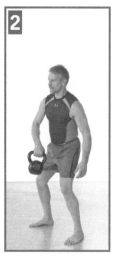 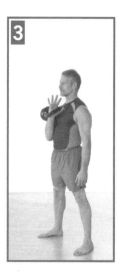 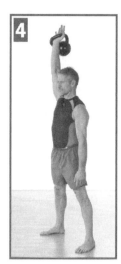 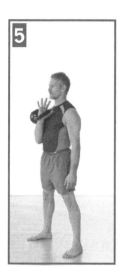

Please note: If you've done barbell cleans, the rack position is NOT the same. Rack position with a kettlebell means the elbow is in tight against the ribs and the wrist is straight but relaxed. Never catch the clean in the palm or fingers—you'll damage your wrists

4 With the kettlebell in the rack position and properly positioned in your hand, grab the ground with your toes and tighten everything all the way up to your shoulder—stay tight the whole time you're pressing and when you bring it back to rack position. Flare your lat and flex your triceps (they should touch) and press straight up. When your arm is fully extended and your elbow is locked out, your biceps should be in line or slightly behind your ear. Your hand should be directly above your shoulder and your palm should be facing to the left or slightly forward. Your shoulder must remain in its socket, not elevated, or you'll injure it.

5 Pull the bell back down using your lat; it should feel like you're doing a pull-up. You should be back in perfect rack position.

To get the bell back to the floor, reverse the motion. Keeping the thumb side of your hand pointing to the center of your body, tip your elbow up and let the bell roll off the inner part of your forearm. As it does so, straighten your arm smoothly, allowing your knees to bend and your hips to sink down to slow the bell's descent to the floor. The descent should be smooth and soft; the bell should lightly kiss the floor, not bang into it. If you feel it jerking your elbow or shoulder, the timing between the bell falling and your knees and hips sinking is off, or you aren't straightening your elbow quickly enough (that is, the bell is moving off your forearm and into your thumb/forefinger grip more quickly than your elbow is straightening).

DETERMINING YOUR CURRENT LEVEL

With the DCP, the amount of weight you can use is limited by how much you can press overhead. Most men should be able to press the 16k (35-lb.) kettlebell but many women may be unable to press the 8k (17-lb.). If you've done overhead pressing with dumbbells, you'll have a good idea of what size kettlebell you can press. Because dumbbells are available in 5-pound increments, you may not be able to find a kettlebell that is near the same weight as the dumbbell. For instance, you may be able to press a 20-pound dumbbell but the closest kettlebell equivalent would be 8k (17-lb.) or 10k (22-lb.). If you're at a gym that is well stocked with kettlebells, you should be able to find the right weight for you.

As you're learning the dead clean portion of the lift, you'll quickly figure out the right weight. Too light and it'll fly up if you pull too hard, too heavy and you won't be able to rack it without a struggle. With the press, the right size should be a moderate intensity level for the Spartan Warrior Workout. Again, the workout calls for a 16k bell for men and a 12k for women so that's what you should be trying to train with. If it's too heavy, drop down one size; if it's too light, go up one. When you do the Spartan workout at full speed, you'll be able to blast through the 25 DCP on each arm easily. You should be able to dead clean a lot more than you can press.

ASSISTANCE EXERCISES

If you've never done the dead clean and press before, you'll want to practice each component separately. Once you can properly dead clean the bell and can perform the press with good form, combine the movements into the dead clean and press.

Dead clean assistance exercises include squats and partial jumps similar to box jumps. The movements are very similar and differ more in range of motion than anything else.

Assistance Exercises for the Dead Clean

SANDBAG SHOULDER

1–2 With the bag on the floor by your feet, grab the front of the bag with your left hand and the rear with your right. Rip it off the floor, using your legs as much as possible. If you need to, dip under the bag as it comes up.

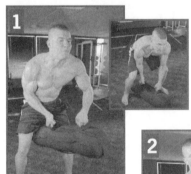

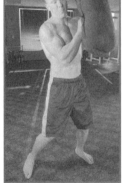

3 As the bag comes up, slip your left hand out from under the bag and wrap your left arm around it. Your right hand will stay on the bag.

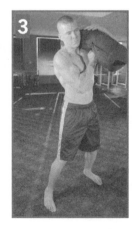

Squats

There are three typical ways of squatting with a kettlebell: the goblet squat, the sumo squat and the racked squat. In all three, the difference is in how you hold the bell. The mechanics are the same as in a bodyweight squat, which we'll look at first.

BODYWEIGHT SQUAT

Follow these directions when doing any type of weighted squat in which the weight is in front of you. The mechanics are much different than squatting with a barbell on your back.

1 Start with your feet about shoulder-width apart and turned outward just a little, no more than 30 degrees. Reach your hands out in front of you at shoulder height; this helps with balance.

2 Activating your hip flexors, push your hips down and back, keeping your shins vertical as your knees bend. Your weight should be on the mid-portion of your foot, back to your heel and also along the outside edge of your feet—think "heels down, instep up." Once at the bottom, stay tight and drive back up through your feet, maintaining the heels-down, instep-up foot position. Don't bounce out of the bottom; it will cause you to lose control and it allows your core to deactivate.

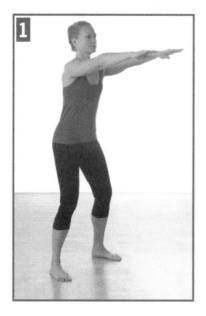

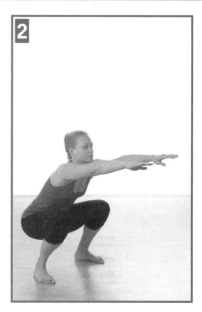

USING YOUR HIP FLEXORS

To feel what it's like to pull with your hip flexors, lie on your back, bend your knees 90 degrees, lift your feet off the floor and point your toes up. Have your partner grab the tops of your feet and pull them with about 5 percent of their strength. Resist their pull—you should feel the area above your hip joint activate. Now stand up and squat using those same muscles to pull yourself down.

GOBLET SQUAT

This is so named because someone thought the kettlebell looked like a big goblet when held upside down in both hands.

1 Hold the bell with both hands by its "horns" at sternum level. The bell will be close to your body but not touching, and your elbows should be down.

2 Keeping your torso upright, squeeze your abs and pull yourself down with your hip

flexors. Try to get your hips below your knees if possible, but don't compromise your structure by tipping over, letting your knees collapse or otherwise losing form. If you have the flexibility in your hips and lower back, try to get your butt to your calves. Squat as deeply as your ability allows. With practice and stretching, you'll get better.

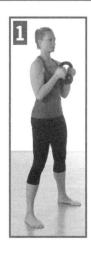
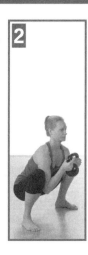

FRONT SQUAT

The mechanics for the front squat are the same as those for the goblet squat, except you're holding the bell in rack position. Your body will move away from your forearm and hand as it descends—the arm itself doesn't move in and out. When you stand up, your body will move back against your arm.

1 Start with the bell in the rack position (elbow is in tight against the ribs, wrist is straight but relaxed, forearm is leaning slightly inward toward the body).

2 Keeping your torso upright, squeeze your abs and pull yourself down with your hip flexors. Try to get your hips below your knees if possible, but don't compromise your structure by tipping over, letting your knees collapse or otherwise losing form.

If you have the flexibility in your hips and lower back, try to get your butt to your calves. Squat as deeply as your ability allows. With practice and stretching, you'll get better.

Perform reps on both sides.

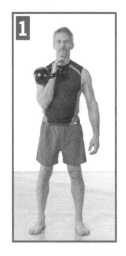

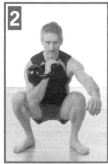

The sumo squat takes its name from the Japanese sumo wrestler's wide stance. Because the bell stops you when it touches the floor, your squat depth won't be nearly as deep as with a goblet squat or a front squat. Your squat depth will also vary depending on the size of the bell.

1 Start with the bell on the floor between your feet, which are a bit more than shoulder-width apart. Grab the bell with both hands by the handle, keeping your torso upright and sinking your hips down and back. Your arms must be straight here; don't squat deeper than is necessary to reach the handle with straight arms.

2 Drive your heels into the floor, lead with your shoulders and straighten your knees as your hips move forward. As with all squats, your butt shouldn't come up before your shoulders do.

3 Sink your hips down and back a little to return the bell to the floor between your feet. Remember to keep your torso up throughout the movement. This is a squatting movement so you should feel this mostly in the quads. If you feel this in your hamstrings and glutes, you're pushing your hips back too far and doing a sumo deadlift.

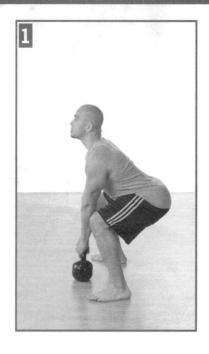

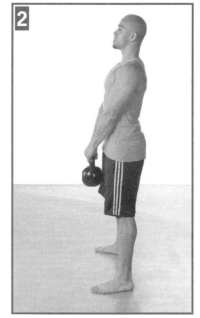

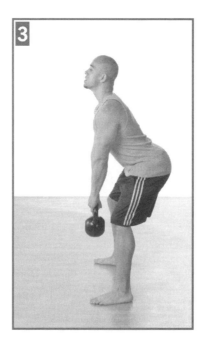

H2H SUMO SQUAT

The hand switch is the same as in the H2H Sumo Deadlift (page 65), while the hip movement is the same as the Sumo Squat.

1–2 Start with the bell on the floor between your feet. Hold the bell in one hand and stand straight up quickly, extending your hips. The momentum will cause the bell to continue rising a little at the top and your elbow will bend slightly because of it.

3 Quickly switch hands and squat back down, kissing the floor with the bell. Do not resist the downward force with your arm; your elbow should be straight as the bell touches the floor. If you feel any discomfort in your elbow, you're doing something wrong.

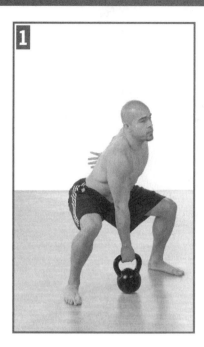

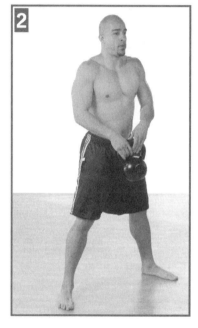

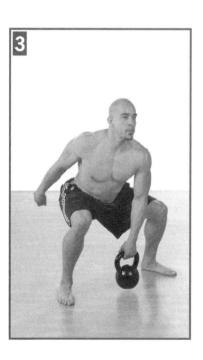

JUMP SQUAT

Jump squats should first be performed with body weight alone. Later, you may be ready to add extra weight. In learning to jump you must also learn to land. Improper landing technique will jar the body and can wreck your knees and lower back. To start, we'll do jumps without leaving the ground to practice the landing.

1–2 Stand with your feet about shoulder-width apart and pointed forward or turned out slightly. Staying flat-footed, pull yourself down as deep as you can go without leaning forward. Push your arms down hard behind you to give you extra power.

3 Explode upward but keep your toes on the floor as your hips fully extend (note: photo shows full squat jump). Once fully extended, sink your hips back and down, letting your knees bend, and sink back onto your heels or as deep as you can go, the same as the initial squat in steps 1–2. Be graceful and soft—no jarring of the body.

Once you've mastered that, you can jump off the floor, keeping your legs fairly straight and your feet just a few inches off the floor. Use the same soft landing. Make contact with the balls of your feet first, then sink back onto your heels as your hips sink down, dropping back into a deep squat; repeat without pausing.

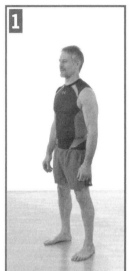
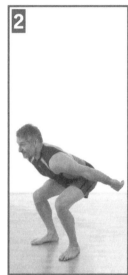
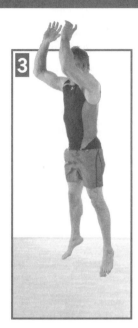

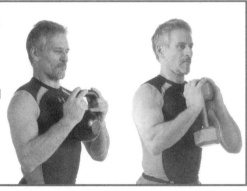

VARIATION: Holding the kettlebell or dumbbell in your hands, drop into a quarter squat and jump as high as you can. Land softly, sink back into the quarter squat and repeat.

JUMP TUCK

The progression after a jump squat is a jump tuck. This is a very powerful hip movement.

1–2 Using minimal knee bend to initiate the movement, jump as high as you can and forcefully and quickly bring your knees to your chest. Remember to keep the landing soft.

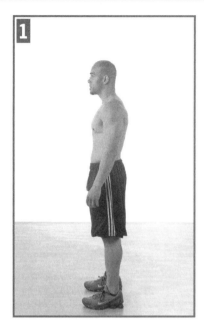

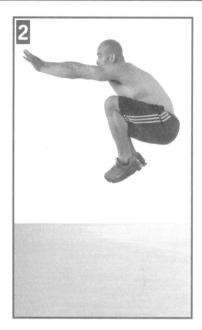

OVERHEAD SQUAT

Some people teach a rotation in the hips as you go into the overhead squat. This lets you get deeper but changes the nature of the movement. In our case, we're trying to improve shoulder range of motion. If your shoulders, mid-back or lower back are tight, you won't be able to squat very deeply before your arm moves from the vertical position.

1 Stand and press the bell overhead, keeping your elbow locked and your shoulder packed.

2 Look straight ahead and squat down, keeping your arm vertical. Don't go deeper than your shoulder allows.

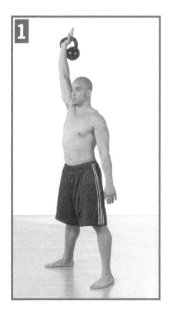

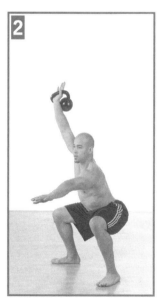

SANDBAG CLEAN TO PRESS

1–2 Hold the bag by its ends with your palms facing each other, parallel to your hips. Rip the bag up, keeping it close to your body.

3 As it reaches shoulder height, let the bag roll over your hands and drive it overhead.

Drop it back to the floor and repeat.

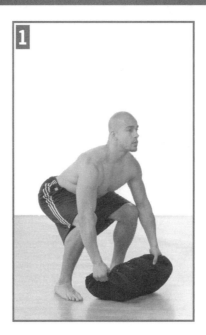

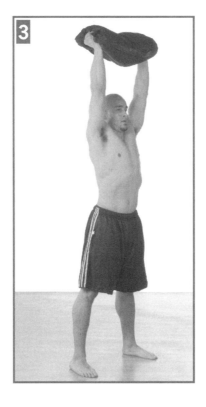

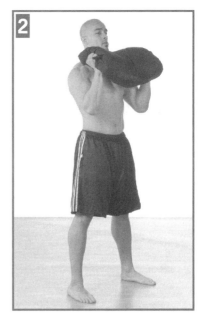

Windmills

Windmills are an awesome movement. Depending on whether you have the weight overhead, are lifting it from the floor or both, the windmill will tax your muscles in many new and different ways, all of which will make you stronger and more flexible, and will improve mobility as well as create a stronger core and shoulder. While doing the windmill, you may feel a stretch in one or both hamstrings; if you bend your knees you lose the stretch. Bending the un-weighted knee (which, in the example below, would be the left) tends to shift your weight away from your supporting right leg and can put more strain on your back.

At first, we'll practice this with no weight. As you get better at it, we'll add weight on the bottom, then we'll move the weight overhead, and finally we'll use the weight top and bottom. Some notes to remember when doing a windmill:

- Keep a long spine throughout the movement.

- Keep the knees straight but not locked.

- Don't shift your weight to the opposite side.

- Don't bend the back—push the hips.

- Don't rotate the back.

- Keep the upper arm totally vertical. Don't let it drift to the side.

- Look up at the upper arm throughout the entire movement to help keep it fixed in space, except when you're standing totally upright.

- Do let the upper arm rotate at the shoulder. The right hand rotates counter-clockwise, the left clockwise.

Once they're folded, many people reach the point where they're at maximum depth because of flexibility issues then bend through their spine to put their hand on the floor. Don't do this. You'll get hurt if you do this with a weight overhead.

1 Stand with your feet about shoulder-width apart and raise your right hand straight up. Turn your left foot toward the left about 45 degrees; your right foot should point straight ahead.

2 Keeping both knees straight, push your hip hard to the right. There should be a straight line from your right hand through your body, into your right leg and into the floor; your left hand should be against your left inner thigh. Fold over through your left hip; do NOT rotate your hips or waist. Make sure you aren't bending your spine as you go lower. Your right arm must remain vertical but allow it to rotate away from you as you go lower. Your left hand should follow the inside of your left leg to keep your shoulders and hips in the same plane. Stop when you feel your knees bend.

Squeeze your glutes and abs hard to stand tall, following the same path you went down. Switch sides.

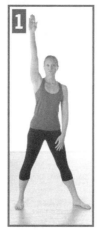
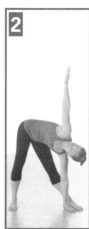

LOW WINDMILL

1 Stand with your feet about shoulder-width apart and raise your right hand straight up as though you just pressed the dumbbell or kettlebell. Hold a weight in your left hand. Turn your left foot toward the left about 45 degrees; your right foot should point straight ahead.

2 Push your hip to the right and fold over your left hip; keep looking up at your right hand. Go as deeply as possible without bending your knees or your spine.

Once you've reached your maximum depth, squeeze hard and pull yourself up.

Don't go heavy until you have it down.

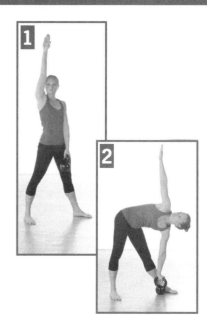

OVERHEAD WINDMILL

It's critical that the upper arm stays vertical in this movement.

Caution: During the overhead windmill, you must be ready to bail out if necessary. If you lose control, let the weight fall and run the other way!

1 Stand with your feet about shoulder-width apart and press a light kettlebell or dumbbell up. Keep your arm vertical.

2 Push your hip out hard to the right and let your shoulder rotate (right arm rotates counter-clockwise, left rotates clockwise). Slide your left hand down the inside of your left leg. When either knee starts to bend, your spine

bends, or your left hand reaches the floor, pause briefly and stay tight.

Use your abs and glutes to pull yourself back up to a standing position looking forward. As you come up, let your shoulder rotate back to its starting position.

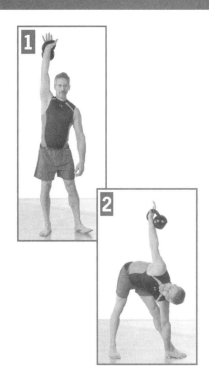

DOUBLE WINDMILL

This combines the low and overhead windmills. The bell in the lower hand will prevent you from going as deeply so don't expect as much of a stretch in the hamstrings as with the overhead-only version; however, the abs will take a tremendous amount of stress.

1–2 Perform the windmill using a lighter weight overhead and a heavier one in the lower hand. Keep your spine straight and long. Follow the steps outlined in both the overhead and low windmill, staying focused on the overhead arm.

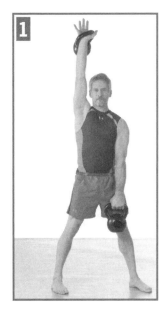
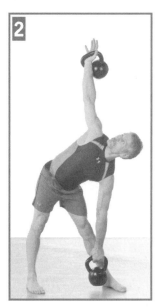

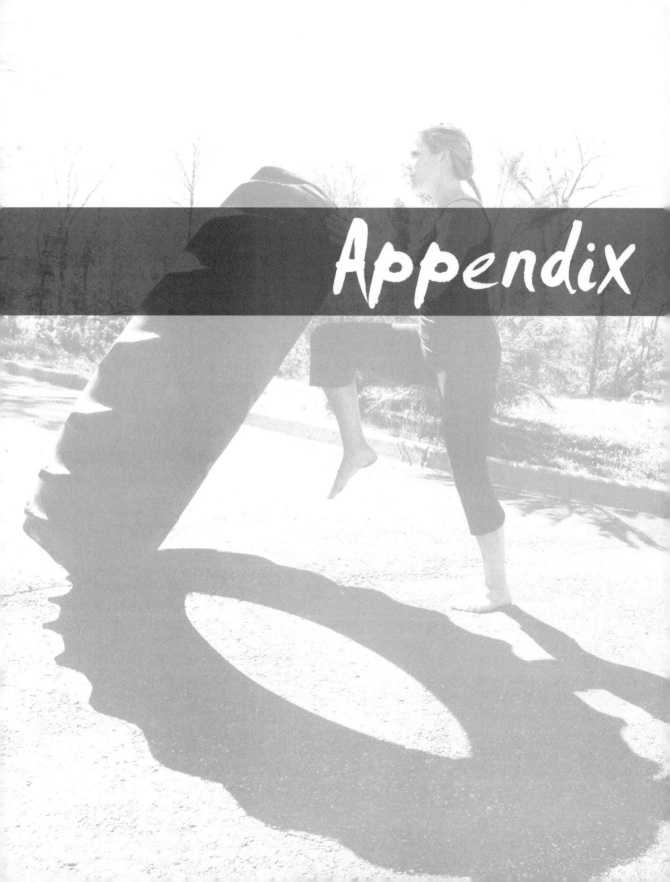

Appendix

General Physical Preparedness

General physical preparedness (GPP) is really about how "in shape" you are and is the lowest level of athleticism. For people who play sports, amateur or pro, GPP represents the foundation upon which they build their technical proficiencies, tactics and strategies and learn to tie everything together.

Without a good GPP foundation, you'll run out of gas while working on more sport-specific tasks or during the actual game or competition. For example, a boxer who lasts only three rounds before getting tired and slowing down needs to focus more on his GPP. A boxer who is getting beat to the punch or has slower footwork than his opponent needs to work on better hand speed or footwork through technique practice, like hitting the speed bag, or working with his coach on timing.

Because the Spartan workout is not focused on one thing, it's really a GPP workout, but you still need skill (good form and technique) to perform it quickly and safely. To augment the six primary exercises, we've incorporated some GPP-specific exercises into the program design to ramp up your overall stamina. These include jump rope, sledgehammer work, tire flipping, sled pulling and pushing as well as mountain climbers and burpees. These exercises are to improve your conditioning level but are also used to improve your ability in many of the six main exercises. Some equipment you'll need:

Tractor tire: A heavy tractor tire (150–250 lb.) can help you create phenomenal power in your lower body. If you don't have one handy, you can get a used tire free from a tractor or heavy equipment supply store. Most people, even smaller women, should be able to handle the 150-pound tire; however, if you're severely deconditioned, you may want to go down to a 100-pound tire. The height of the tire will be about five or six feet.

Sledgehammer: An 8- or 10-pound sledgehammer from your local hardware store will help you build upper body strength. There are heavier ones, but learn the technique and get used to the movement before going too heavy. You'll be pounding on a tractor tire or, if more readily available, a log that's about 18 inches high and at least 12 inches in diameter.

Sled: You can buy a pulling sled from several fitness sales sites on the web or you can use an old disc-type of sled used for snow sledding. You'll need some sort of heavy strapping or webbing, typically tie-down straps, which you can purchase from most hardware stores. If your sled doesn't have a place to attach the webbing to, you can drill a hole and put an eye bolt through the sled, loop the webbing through the eye bolt and grab each end in a hand. The surface you pull on will affect the sled and how it slides.

Resistance bands: Using strong resistance bands such as those from jumpstretch.com or ironwoody.com adds a new dimension to your training. You can do all kinds of exercises with them and create variable resistance when using barbells or doing pull-ups and push-ups. You can also use bands instead of kettlebells or dumbbells for many exercises; the variable resistance of the bands works your body differently than using a fixed weight. They're also portable so you can use them anywhere. In the Spartan Warrior Workout, we'll use them mainly for help in doing pull-ups.

Jump rope: You don't need to spend a lot on a jump rope; the cheap plastic ones will do fine for our purposes. If you decide to spend more time working on jump rope technique (doing double-unders and other advanced rope movements), you might invest in a more-expensive rope. Whichever rope you choose should be 9 to 10 feet long, depending on your height. If you're short, you'll need to tie some knots in it near the handles so it isn't too long.

1 With the tire flat on the ground, squat down deeply with your chest touching the tire and your hips down. Hook your fingers underneath, preferably gripping the tread.

2–3 Lead with your shoulders and drive forward; extend your hips and stand. Use your legs, not your arms. As you stand, flip your hands from face up to palms forward. You may have to bump the tire with a knee during the transition phase for some added lift. Once you've switched your grip, drive through and push it over.

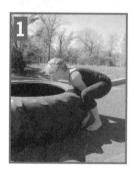
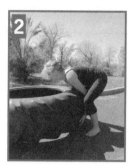
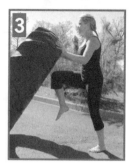

TIRE JUMP VARIATION: To further work the legs, you can also jump in and out of the tire.

Tire flipping requires you to use your entire body in a coordinated way and will make both your deadlifts and squats stronger.

JUMP ROPE

Jumping rope combines aerobic work with hand and foot coordination, but once you get the hang of it, it's like doing a long run—you have to really crank out the reps to get good results from your efforts.

If you've never jumped rope, practice by trying to do 100 jumps without stopping or missing. Once you can do 100, start jumping for time. Try to do 150 reps in 1 minute. As your technique improves and your legs get stronger, you'll be able to go faster and longer. You should be able to jump for 5 minutes at a time in a few weeks, averaging 125 to 150 jumps per minute.

Increase the difficulty with light ankle weights, a weighted vest or wrist weights but be careful— they'll move around and bang hard.

1 Hold a handle in each hand; keep your hands at about your waist line. The rope movement comes from the wrists, not the arms, so try to keep your elbows stationary. With the rope behind you, use your wrists to whip it over your head. As it comes down toward your feet, jump just high enough (an inch or so) to let the rope pass under your feet. The jumping is done with the calves and the balls of the feet; you'll never be flat footed when jumping rope.

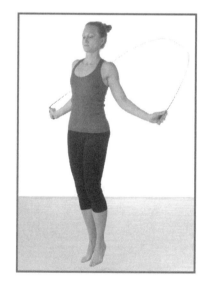

SLEDGEHAMMER

Pounding a tire or a log with a sledgehammer will improve your endurance, work your core and strengthen your shoulders and back. If you're hitting a log, you'll have to learn to absorb the shock and keep a solid grip or it will sting your hands and the shock wave will travel back up your arm. Don't miss your target; many people have banged their shins or knees up because they lost focus and missed.

1 Stand with your feet about shoulder-width apart. Hold the sledgehammer to your lower right side; your right hand will be near the head of the sledgehammer, your left hand will be a few inches from the bottom of the handle.

2–3 Circle the sledgehammer down to the right a little then behind, up and over your right shoulder.

4 As the sledgehammer starts to come down, let your right hand slide down the handle so it ends up close to your left hand. At the same time sink your hips down and slam the sledgehammer into the tire. Be careful—it may bounce back! At the point of impact, tighten your grip or the sledgehammer will twist out of your hands.

You may now either do the right side again by sliding your right hand back up toward the head and moving the sledge to right rear again, or you can switch to a left-handed grip. Bring it to left rear, circling it back then up and over your left shoulder.

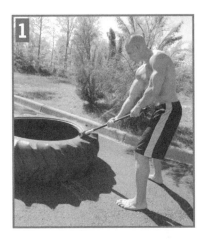

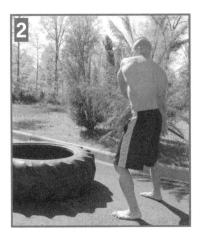

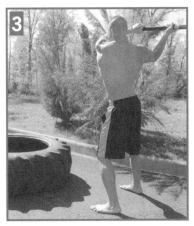

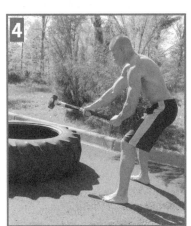

VARIATION: Occasionally you'll assume a staggered stance, with your right foot forward and left behind or vice versa. If your right foot is forward, you'll hit with a left-hand grip (left hand closer to the head); if your left foot is forward, you'll use a right-hand grip. The non-dominant grip will feel weird and you won't have nearly as much power or coordination for a while.

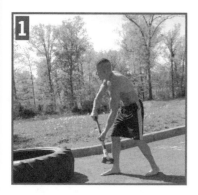 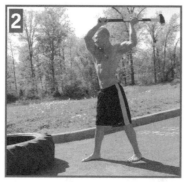 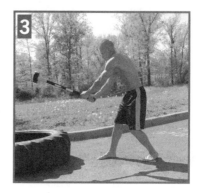

MOUNTAIN CLIMBERS

With mountain climbers, your upper body is constantly under a dynamic load and your legs are always moving. In addition, you need a strong core and hip flexors. Your hips should not go up and down or rock from side to side. Keep your butt down!

1 Assume a good high plank position and bring one knee up under you. You'll be supporting your weight with your upper body throughout the movement. Keep your elbows locked and hands shoulder-width apart.

2–3 Switch feet by quickly driving the knee that's under you back and pull the other knee up. Your feet should not slide along the floor. The only time your feet touch is the split second when one knee is up under you and the other leg is fully extended; as soon as you hit that position, move right through it and keep going.

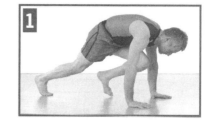

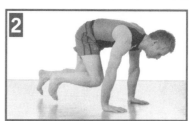

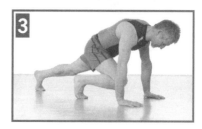

SLED PULL

Sled pulling and pushing are great ways to finish your workout and should be done as heavy as possible.

1 With your arms behind you at about hip level, stay tight and start walking forward. You'll have to dig in hard to pull heavy, driving with the balls of your feet. Don't try to pull with your arms. This really hits the quads hard!

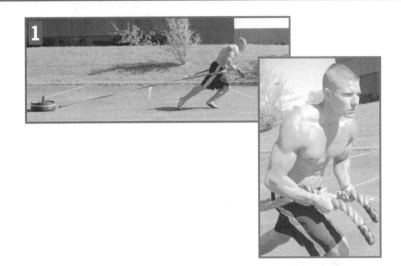

SLED PUSH

When pushing, keep your abs tight and your back flat. Your hands should be about shoulder-width apart and your elbows straight but not hyper-extended. Bending your elbows makes your chest work harder, but you can't generate as much force. Keeping your elbows straight allows the force to move from the ground, through your body and out your arms, keeping the work to the posterior chain (your backside).

If you can't get a hold of a sled you can also use a car or truck; just push on a flat surface and have someone in the vehicle to apply the brakes when needed.

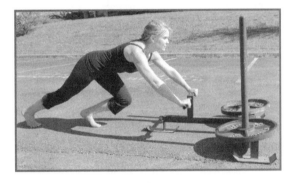

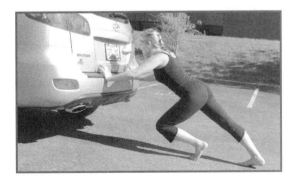

BURPEES

Burpees are a killer GPP exercise; almost anyone can do a version of them. Burpees combine a squat, a push-up or plank, a double-knee tuck and potentially a jump squat.

LEVEL 1

1   Squat and put your hands on the floor.

2–3 Kick both feet back so you're in a solid push-up/high plank position. Try to keep your hips low.

4   Bring both knees back under you and shift from the balls of your feet to a flat foot position and stand. Upon standing, squat back down and repeat.

Stick with level 1 until you're moving your feet at the same time both out and in.

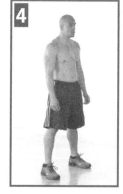

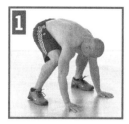
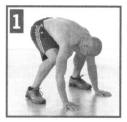
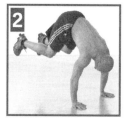
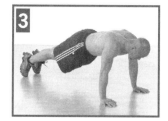

LEVEL 2

For level 2, instead of standing at the end, jump up and reach for the sky. Land softly by absorbing into your legs and go right back to the floor. Your feet should make little to no noise; don't "stick" the landing like they do in gymnastics.

When you can keep your hips motionless while bringing your knees under, add the push-up (level 3).

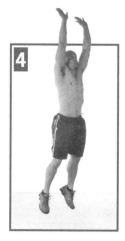

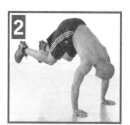
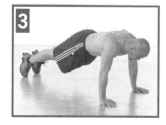

LEVEL 3

For level 3, do a push-up after you come to plank position.

If you can't do a full push-up, do a partial push-up going halfway down, then as you fatigue start doing them on your knees. Instead of jumping for the sky like you did in level 2, just shift back to standing.

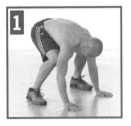
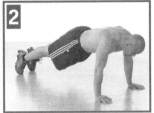
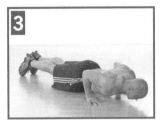
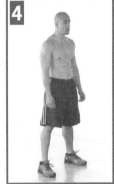

LEVEL 4

Level 4 is very advanced—you need to be able to do 20 or 30 good push-ups without rest before attempting this variation, where you fall into the bottom of a push-up. Once you've gotten to the bottom, push yourself up, then bring the knees back under, return to the flat-foot squat and stand.

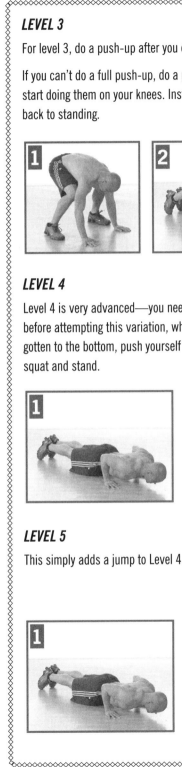
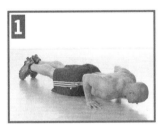
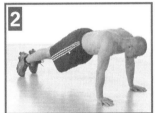
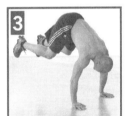
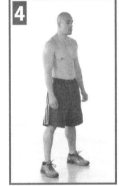

LEVEL 5

This simply adds a jump to Level 4. This will kick your butt!

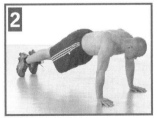
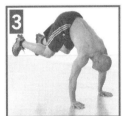
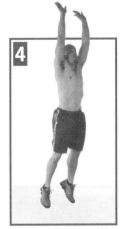

FARMER'S WALK

1 Pick up two heavy bells just like you did in the Suitcase Deadlift (page 63). Stand tall, keep your shoulders in their sockets and walk. Make sure not to lean forward—keep your chest up and shoulders back at all times.

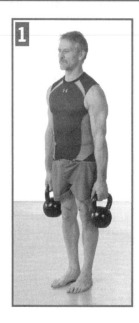

KETTLEBELL RACK WALK

1 Bring one kettlebell to rack position (see page 97) and walk with it for the prescribed distance/time. Switch sides.

VARIATION: This can also be done with two kettlebells.

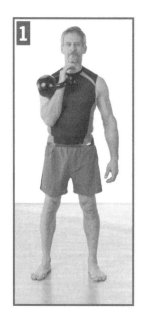

BAND PUSH-UP

Using bands for push-ups is another good way to improve your strength. You can do your push-ups inclined, declined, flat, on your knees or any other variation. Use as heavy a band as you can while maintaining perfect form.

1–2 Place the band in one hand, bring it over and across your shoulder blades, and place the other end in the other hand. Do your push-ups.

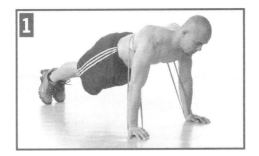

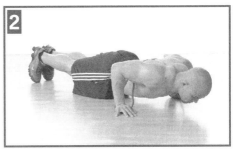

BAND ROW

You can do this with both arms working together or alternating. Mix it up.

1 Attach the band(s) to a sturdy post, a squat rack or even a tree, then step about two feet away from the attachment site.

2 Facing the attachment, use your lats to pull the bands back to your hips in a rowing motion.

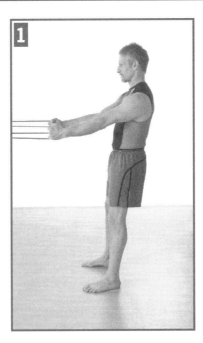

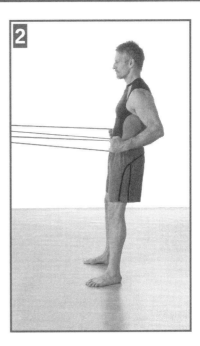

BAND DEADLIFT

You'll want to wear shoes for this.

1 Stand on the band with your feet at least shoulder-width apart. Keep slack in the band between your feet; you don't need tension there.

2 Grasp the band with both hands, push your hips back and bend your knees.

3 Straighten your knees and extend your hips. Stand up tall just as though you were using a barbell.

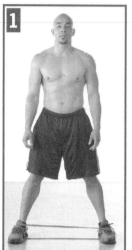
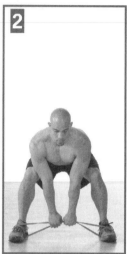
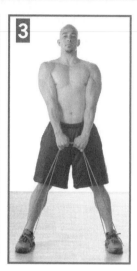

BAND PRESS

This is like doing a bench press or push-up. You can do one arm at a time or both.

1 Wrap the band around your back and grip an end in each hand. Start with your elbows against your ribs, by your sides.

2 Push the ends of the band out from your hips to about chest height.

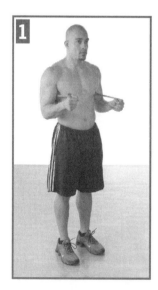
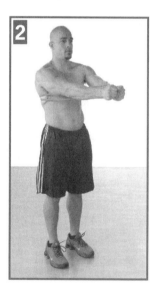

VARIATION: This can also be done by attaching the band(s) to a sturdy post, a squat rack or even a tree.

OVERHEAD STATIC HOLD

1 Lock out one bell overhead and hold for the prescribed amount of time. Switch sides.

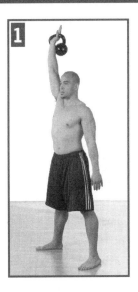

VARIATION: The static hold can also be done with a barbell.

WALKING VARIATION: With the bell(s) locked out overhead, start walking for the prescribed distance/time. Switch sides if you're using one bell.

AB ROLLOUT

The ab wheel, available at most sporting goods stores, will give you rock-solid abs and teach you how to really use your core in everything you do.

1 Kneel on the floor (with a yoga mat under your knees for padding if you wish) and hold the axle of the wheel in each hand.

2 Keeping your abs tight, push from your hips to move forward. Let your arms move ahead of you and keep your head down. To reduce stress on your lower back, keep it rounded, not flat or arched. Go out as far as you can, extending your hips if possible but not letting your thighs touch the floor.

To return to kneeling, stay tight and pull back with your hips; avoid jerking with your arms to get them back under you and keep your chin slightly tucked under.

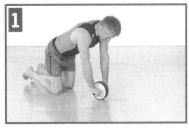

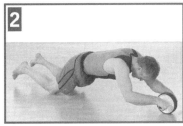

VARIATION: If you can do at least five full ab rollouts from your knees, try starting from your feet. This is much harder—move slowly and stay tight or you'll do a face-plant. Another option is to roll out as far as you can from standing then drop to your knees, finish the rollout then reverse by pulling back to the low start position and finish by lifting your hips and pulling the rest of the way back in.

Warm-Ups, Cool-Downs

Proper warm-up and cool-down movements should be incorporated into every workout you do, and many of the movements should be done on a daily basis, even if you don't train that day.

Warm-ups should be dynamic in nature and mimic the movements that will be performed in the main workout. For example, do light jogging as a warm-up for sprints, or jumping jacks to warm up the arms and legs and to increase the heart rate and blood flow to the extremities. Performing light, easy, bodyweight squats will move blood through the legs and loosen the glutes, hamstrings and quads. Sequences can be crafted that combine various movement patterns into a fluid routine lasting two or three minutes.

Cool-down exercises (which include yoga and general stretching but may also feature certain types of qi gong designed to restore depleted energy and rebuild damaged tissue) should be done to compensate for the movements you did during your primary workout. (Any time you're sore after a workout, it's because you've created micro-tears in the muscle fibers. The muscles rebuild and get stronger to prevent further tearing, hence the need for adequate protein intake.) For instance, if you did a lot of deadlifts, you'd want to focus on movements that keep the hamstrings long as well as open up the outer hips (the piriformis) and the hip flexors, among others. Doing a lot of push-ups or bench presses? Focus on yoga postures that open the chest and shoulders and pull the shoulder blades back.

DESK-HAB

If you sit at a desk all day, compensatory movements should include movements that are the opposite of your seated position; neck retraction and sideways movements, shoulder and chest opening, shoulder blade retraction, hip flexor opening, glute and hamstring lengthening are the primary areas needing work. These movements, when done by themselves and not part of a workout, can be considered pre-hab movements. Beyond that you can use foam rollers and tennis balls to reduce or eliminate points of tension in the body or to work the deep ligaments with gentle tugging and rotation of the joints. See the chapter on Pre-Hab starting on page 147.

PAIN: GOOD VS. BAD

Let's take a second to talk about discomfort or pain as it relates to any movement. On a scale from 1 to 10, with 10 being the most excruciating pain you've ever felt, your discomfort during ANY exercise or movement should be a 3 or less. If it goes above a 3, back off until it's below a 3 or stop.

However, you need to realize and identify the difference between pain/discomfort and hard work/muscle fatigue, especially as it relates to the lower back. Most people have weak abs/core, which also means they have a weak back. When they start to exercise vigorously, especially when doing exercises such as a deadlift or kettlebell swings, they'll start to "feel it in their back" and quit because they think they're injuring their back. The lower back muscles are just like all the other muscles in your body—when they're exercised, they get tired; when they get tired they get the "pump" feeling and start to feel weak. For instance, if you do a bunch of biceps curls, your arms would feel like they're about to explode and fall off your body. The same thing occurs in the back, so if you feel that burn and you know you have no back issues, don't freak out—you're making your back stronger, not damaging it.

JOINT MOBILITY

One sequence of movements you should always do is joint mobility exercises. These movements are designed to pump fresh synovial fluid (the stuff that lubricates and feeds the joints) into the joints, push out old stale fluids and remove mineral deposits that build up over time if we don't move. (That's why your joints feel old and creaky when you sit still for a long time. The joints literally stiffen up because there's no fluid being pushed in.) Doing these movements prime the pump and get the body ready for more vigorous exercise.

Typically we start with the neck, then move to the shoulders and elbows. The wrists can also be done, but we usually move on to the waist due to time constraints. From the waist we move into the low back, then lower into the pelvis. Finally we work the knees. As with the wrists, the ankles can be done if you have time.

As you perform these movements, stay relaxed and breathe normally: exhale as your body moves in on itself, inhale as the body opens. This may feel a little odd at first but you'll get used to it quickly.

The number of reps done all depends on how you feel. If 5 reps of a movement feels good, then 5 it is; if 20 reps feel good, do 20. The only drill I recommend keeping low in reps is the Back Extension Circles (page 130), especially if you have back issues. You may not be able to do them at all; check with your doctor if you're unsure if you should do this or any other movement, stretches or exercises in this book.

Joint Mobility

NECK: SIDE-TO-SIDE ROTATION

1 Stand tall with your arms by your sides.

2 Gently turn your head as far to one side as you can. Lead with your eyes and don't let your shoulders move. Each time try to go a little farther. You may hear a lot of crunchy things in there, but that's normal; it's the mineral deposits breaking up. As long as you feel no discomfort, keep going.

3 Now slowly rotate your neck back to neutral then on to the other side.

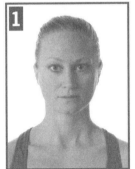
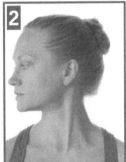
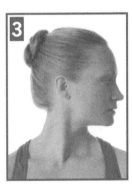

NECK: UP AND DOWN

1 Stand tall with your feet hip-width apart and look straight ahead.

2 Tilt your head back and project your chin up at a 45-degree angle.

3 Lower your chin and project the base of your skull to the sky about 45 degrees up. The goal is to make your vertebrae slide, not just tilt your head.

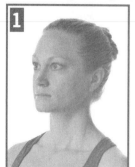
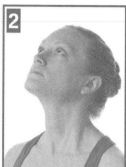
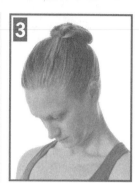

NECK: SIDE-TO-SIDE SLIDE

1 Stand tall with your feet hip-width apart and look straight ahead. Raise your arms and place your index fingers about 1 inch on either side of your head in line with your cheeks. Envision a rod going from one finger to the other and that your head will be sliding along that rod.

2 Keeping your head level (chin parallel to the floor), slide your head to one side and touch that finger. There should be no rotation or tipping of the head. Think of a belly dancer moving her neck side to side but not moving anything else.

3 Slide it to the other side and touch that finger.

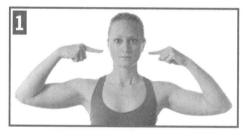
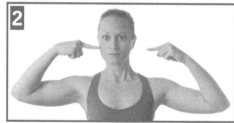
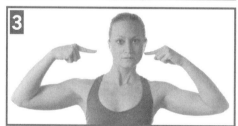

NECK: FRONT-TO-BACK GLIDE

1 Stand tall with your feet hip-width apart, arms relaxed by your sides.

2 Keeping your torso and shoulders locked in place and chin parallel to the floor, slide your chin as far forward as possible. Your chin will angle downward slightly.

3 Pull your head back as far as possible without tipping or turning your head. Focus more on the backward movement than the forward. At this point, your chin should be parallel to the floor.

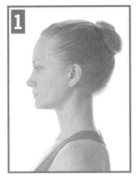
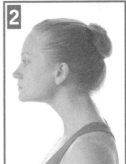
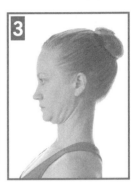

NECK: FIGURE 8

Here your head will trace a sideways figure 8. Try not to turn your head as it goes to the side. At first, keep the side-to-side movement shallow; increase the range of motion as you improve.

1 Stand tall with your feet hip-width apart, arms relaxed by your sides; look straight ahead throughout the exercise.

2 Slide your head forward.

3 With your neck extended, move your head to one side in an arc and continue moving it until it's in the fully retracted position. The movement is a semi-circle.

4 Move your head forward again, moving through the center until your neck is fully extended.

5 Slide to the other side in an arc and bring your head back to the fully retracted position.

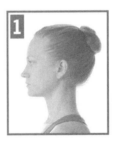
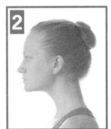
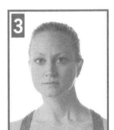

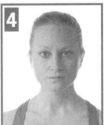
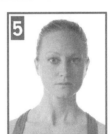

FORWARD/BACKWARD SHOULDER CIRCLES

1 Stand with your feet together and your right hand at your side, palm facing away from your body, elbow straight. Raise your arm up to the rear, leading with your thumb.

2 When your arm is at 12 o'clock, your thumb is facing forward and your palm is to the side.

3 Let your arm continue its motion; when it returns to the start position, externally rotate it again.

When you're ready, reverse the direction by starting with your palm facing your leg and leading the circle with your thumb. Do both sides.

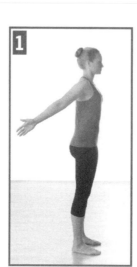
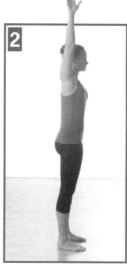
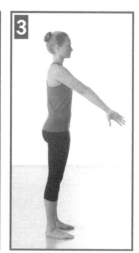

CROSS-BODY ARM CIRCLES

Think of these as if playing an air guitar, Pete Townshend style.

1 Standing with your body facing straight ahead, bring one arm across your body, keeping the elbow straight and the thumb pointing up, palm facing the rear.

2–3 Lift up the arm and bring it over and to the rear, maintaining the same angle in the rear as in the front.

4 Bring the arm under and to the front.

When you're ready, reverse direction. Do both sides.

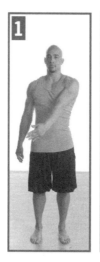
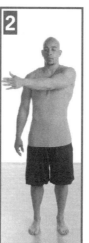
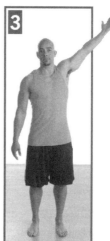
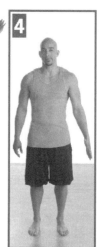

REAR SHOULDER CIRCLES

1 Stand with your feet hip-width apart. Keeping your torso forward, reach back as far as you can with one arm until your triceps touches your lat.

2–3 Moving from your shoulder and keeping your elbow straight, circle your arm behind you.

When you're ready, reverse direction, then switch sides.

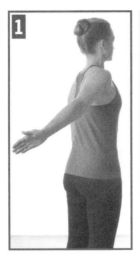
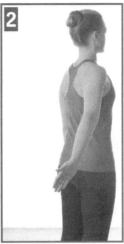
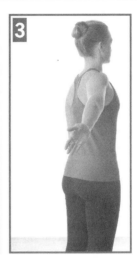

VERTICAL ELBOW CIRCLES

1 Stand with your feet hip-width apart and raise your forearm and upper arm parallel to the floor, keeping your shoulder relaxed and in its socket. Bend your elbow 90 degrees so that your hand is in a loose fist directly in front of your sternum.

2–3 Moving only from your elbow, draw a large circle with your fist, extending your forearm forward and then bringing your fist back toward your sternum. Bend your wrist so that when your elbow is extended, your hand is still in front of your sternum.

When you're ready, reverse direction, then switch sides.

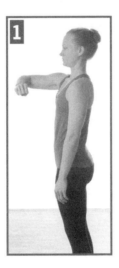
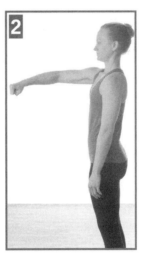
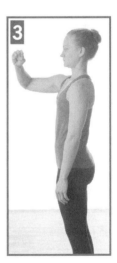

HORIZONTAL ELBOW CIRCLES

1 Stand with your feet hip-width apart and raise your right forearm perpendicular to the floor, keeping your shoulder down and in its socket. Place the back of your left hand under your right elbow and raise your left upper arm parallel to the floor. Make sure your right hand is in line with your right shoulder.

2–3 Moving from your elbow, circle your forearm, drawing a large circle with your fist. Make sure you fully extend your elbow as your fist moves to the front and back around.

When you're ready, switch directions and then switch arms.

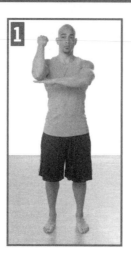
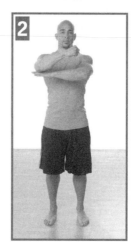
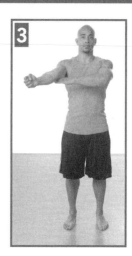

HANGING ELBOW CIRCLES

1 Stand tall with your feet hip-width apart. Raise your arms out to the sides and bend your elbows 90 degrees so that your forearms hang freely toward the floor. If you have tight shoulders, resist the tendency to tilt forward.

2–3 Moving only from your elbows, circle both forearms.

When you're ready, reverse direction.

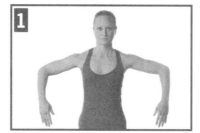
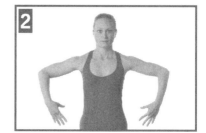
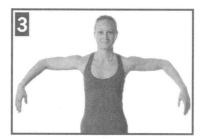

WAIST TWIST

1 Stand with your feet about shoulder-width apart, arms hanging loosely by your sides.

2 Rotate to the right, moving from your waist. Keep your hips and knees facing forward. As your torso turns, move your head with the rest of your spine. Your arms will move by way of momentum. If you're turning toward the right, let your right hand swing around and gently tap the kidney area on the left. Your left hand will rise up and gently touch the area just below your right shoulder.

3 Unwind to the left, letting your arms wrap around.

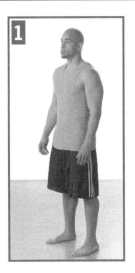
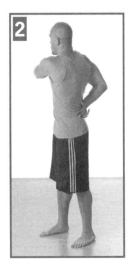
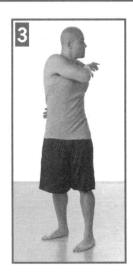

PELVIC CIRCLES

This is a belly dancer's signature movement. If you do this right, you should feel your lower abs. The upper body and shoulder move, but only in counterpoint to the hips. Try to make the movement fluid.

1 Stand tall with your feet hip-width apart and knees slightly bent. Push your pelvis forward.

2–4 Move your hips in a circular fashion to the right side and around to the rear; your hips should be pushed back. Keep moving around to the side and back to the front with your hips pushed forward.

When you're ready, switch directions.

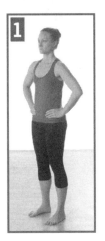
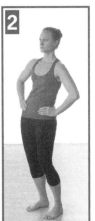
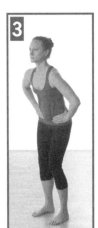
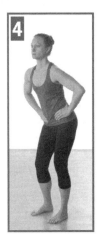

BACK EXTENSION CIRCLES

This movement combines a back bend (extension) with flexion while moving in a circle. The forward flexion should be no more than a 90-degree fold through the hip; the back extension should only be as far back as is comfortable (3 or less on the Rate of Perceived Discomfort scale).

1 Stand with your feet about shoulder-width apart and hands on your hips.

2 Fold at your hips, keeping your chest out and knees soft.

3 Push your hips to the left, shifting your weight to your left leg. Your torso will move to the right and your right knee will bend.

4 Once you've gone as far as you can to the right, roll your torso backward, rotating through your waist, and lift your chest (the sternum specifically) toward the ceiling. Let your head fall back.

5 Move your torso to the left; when you've gone as far as you can, rotate so that your chest is facing the floor and move back to the start position.

When you're ready, reverse the movement.

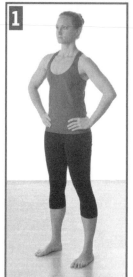
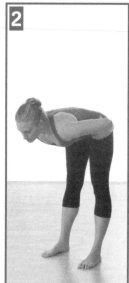
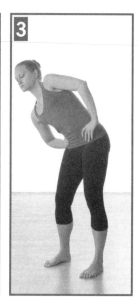
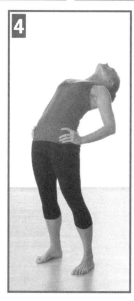
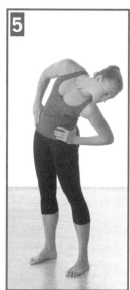

HIP CIRCLES

If you have problems with balance, stand near a wall and just barely touch it with a finger of the hand opposite the side you're working (if you're working your left side, use your right hand). After a few sessions, you'll find you no longer need the wall. It also helps to gaze softly at a spot about 10 feet out on the floor in front of you.

1 Stand tall with your feet hip-width apart.

2 Stand on your left leg and bring your right leg up, bending your knee 90 degrees; your thigh should be parallel to the floor.

3–4 Rotate your hip so that the inside part of your foot points upward. Keeping your knee bent throughout the movement, move your right leg as far to the right as possible.

5–6 Lower it to the right rear. As you lower it, your hip will rotate back in.

7 Bring it up from the right rear to the left front, with your thigh parallel to the floor. At this point, your right knee is outside your left thigh and pointing about 45 degrees to the left.

8 Bring your leg back through the starting position and repeat. Make sure to rotate your hip to get the most benefit from this movement.

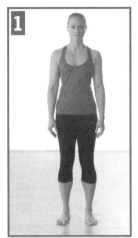

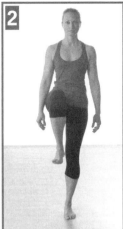

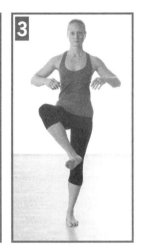

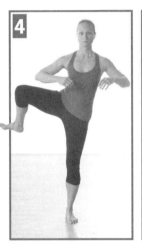

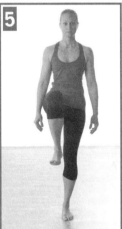

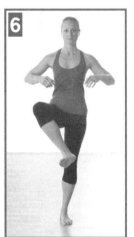

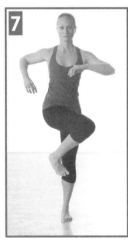

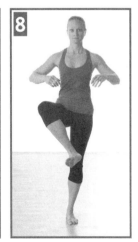

REVERSE HIP CIRCLES

The reverse hip circle also takes some practice.

1 Instead of taking the leg out to the side (right, if we're working the right hip), move the upper leg to the left as far as possible.

2 Keeping the knee bent the whole time, lower it and move it diagonally to the rear.

3 When you've brought it back as far as possible, lift the knee and rotate the hip so that the inner thigh is parallel to the floor.

4 Continue bringing the knee back to the front, rotating the hip so that the top of the thigh is once again parallel to the floor.

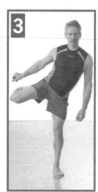
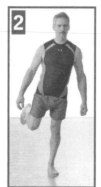
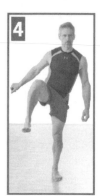

KNEE CIRCLES

1 Stand with your feet together and bend your knees as deeply as you can; place your hands just above your knees on your thighs. Keep your heels on the floor.

2 Circle your knees to the right, straightening them as you do.

3 After 10 reps, circle your knees to the left.

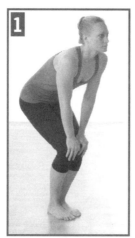
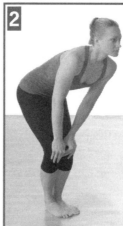
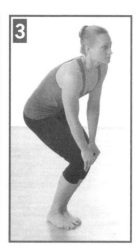

DYNAMIC WARM-UPS

The purpose of the dynamic warm-up is to prepare the body for the main portion of the workout. Typically, the dynamic warm-up should involve the same muscle groups as the main workout, so if the main workout is the deadlift, the warm-up should include some active hamstring and glute work. Squats and lunges done at a moderate pace are another way to get the body moving. The main thing to remember is that these warm-ups are just that: warm-ups. Ease into them, move at a moderate pace, focus on form and get the blood moving through the muscles.

Some people ask why we don't do static stretches like the split stretch or seated hamstring stretch. The reason is because they're static—nothing is being done to warm up the muscles. Also, most static stretching is done to make the muscles relax, with the erroneous belief that you can lengthen the muscles and that by doing so you're preparing the muscles for action. In reality, that's the worst thing you can do for a warm-up. Static stretches, however, are great for a cool-down; doing them then will help to compensate for the tension created by lifting weights.

You can use almost any bodyweight exercise, done for a short period of time, as a warm-up. You can also do light weightlifting as well. The kettlebell swing is a great tool for warm-ups.

For my warm-ups I like to do a 2-minute straight set of 4 exercises done for 30 seconds each. Here's a typical dynamic warm-up:

- Squat Thrust
- Shuffles
- Mountain Climbers
- Jumping Jacks

Here's another:

- Walkouts
- High Knees
- Cross-over Lunge
- Leg Swings (15 seconds/side)

One more with body weight:

- Squat
- Side-to-Side Stretch
- Push-ups
- One-Legged Squat (each leg)
- Plank
- Side Plank (each side)

At 4 minutes, the bodyweight warm-up is a bit longer, but hits all the major muscles, including the abs.

The following uses a kettlebell. Each exercise is done for 30 seconds with no rest in between. As a warm-up, you should use a moderate weight, usually one size down from your normal bell:

- 2-hand swings
- 1-hand swings on the right
- 1-hand swings on the left
- H2H or alternating swings

WALKOUT

1 Stand with your feet hip-width apart.

2 Bend at the waist, trying to keep your knees straight, and put your hands flat on the floor in front of your feet.

3–4 Walk your hands out until you've reached at least a high plank position. Go further if you can but don't let your hips sag.

5 Walk your hands back in. If you wish, you can stand up before walking your hands out again.

> **VARIATION:** You can also add in a push-up when you reach the high plank position.

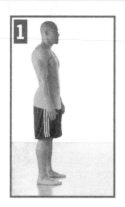
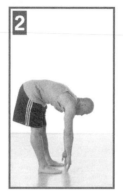
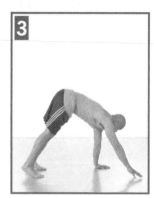
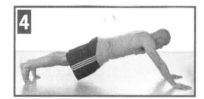
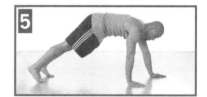

HIGH KNEES

1 Stand tall and hold your hands at chest height, palms facing down.

2–3 Bring one knee up to touch the palm, put it down, then bring the other one up. Don't allow your torso to bend—stay tall and really focus on lifting the knee.

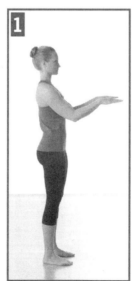
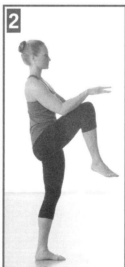
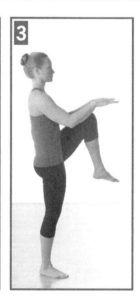

CROSS-OVER LUNGE

1 Stand with your feet hip-width apart.

2–3 Step your left leg behind your right. Keep your hips forward and your torso upright; try to keep your feet on the same line. Sink your knees; your rear knee should be close to your front ankle.

Bring your left leg back under you and stand up. Repeat to the other side.

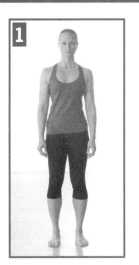
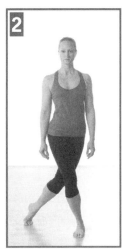
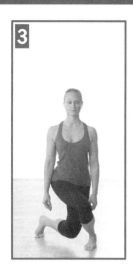

LEG SWINGS

Don't go too high, too hard or too fast with these or you may pull something; ease into them.

1 Stand with your feet hip-width apart and place your hands on your hips.

2 Shift your weight to the right so that your left foot is no longer on the floor. Moving from your hip and keeping your knee straight, swing your leg forward, keeping your toes pulled back.

Let your leg come back down and place it back on the floor—don't let it swing behind you. Stay tall with your chest out. Placing the foot on the floor works quad and hip flexor strength and stretches the hamstrings.

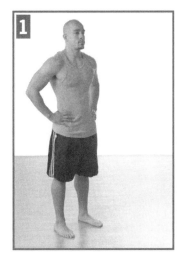
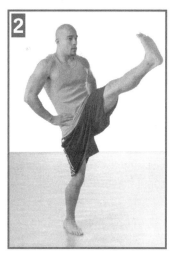

SQUAT THRUST

1 From a standing position, squat down and put your hands on the floor.

2 Drive your feet back so you're in a high plank (top of a push-up).

3 Quickly pull your knees back under you, move back to your squat position and stand up.

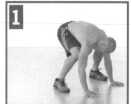
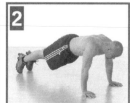
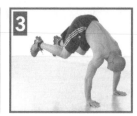

SHUFFLES

1–2 Standing tall, move your feet back and forth under you, quickly switching feet. Try to minimize the up and down movement, but don't just slide your feet on the floor.

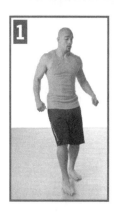
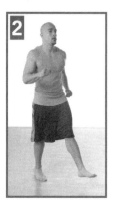

PLANK

See page 54 for more details about the plank.

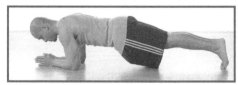

Plank

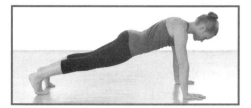

High Plank

MOUNTAIN CLIMBERS

1 Assume a high plank with one knee tucked under you.

2–3 Switch feet by quickly driving the knee that's under you back and pull the other knee up. Your feet should not slide along the floor. The only time your feet touch is the split second when one knee is up under you and the other leg is fully extended; as soon as you hit that position, move right through it and keep going.

Repeat.

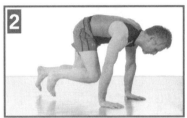

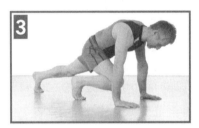

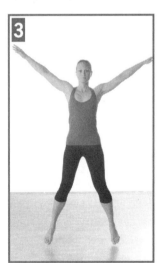

JUMPING JACKS

1 Stand with your feet together and palms facing your legs.

2 Quickly spread your legs to about 1.5 times shoulder-width apart (it should be comfortable without straining your knees) and at the same time bring your arms up the sides and overhead. Try to touch your hands overhead; if you have tight shoulders you may not be able to do this.

3 Bring your feet back together and your arms to your sides. The hands and feet move together and never stop; this is a continual movement.

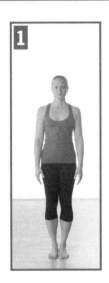

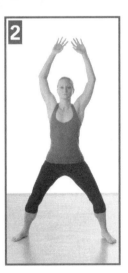

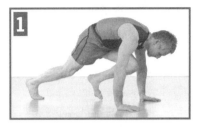

SIDE-TO-SIDE STRETCH

When you shift to the sides, make sure the knee points in the same direction as the foot. This is an inner thigh stretch, NOT a lunge.

1 Take a wide stance, about 1.5 to 2 times shoulder-width apart, with hips and torso facing forward and feet flat on the floor.

2 Shift your weight to the left, bend your left knee and let your left foot rotate about 45 degrees to the left. Turn your right foot a little to the left. Don't rotate through the waist; keep your torso forward. Sink your hips down but don't bend over; stay tall. Try to get the thigh of your working (bent) leg parallel to the floor.

Switch sides.

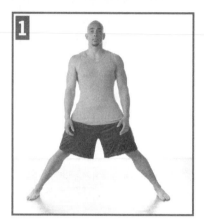
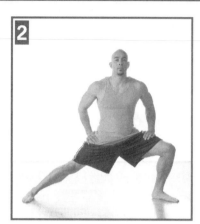

ONE-LEGGED SQUAT

This is the same movement pattern as a regular squat, but it's NOT a full-depth pistol; it's a partial range-of-motion squat done on one leg.

1 Stand with your feet hip-width apart.

2–3 Raise your left leg up in front of you, keeping your knee straight. Pull yourself down with your right hip flexors, trying to keep your torso upright. Keep your abs tight throughout. Go as low as you can.

Drive through your heel to stand back up.

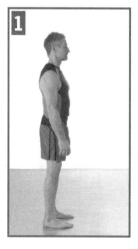
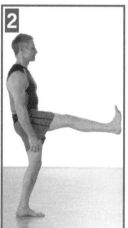
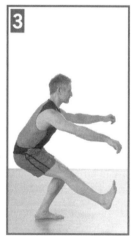

COOL-DOWNS

The goal of the cool-down (or warm-down, as some refer to this phase of the workout) is to release the residual tension caused by resistance training and to let the heart rate and body temperature gradually return to their normal ranges. When you exercise, especially when lifting heavy, your body tightens up in bands across the body, which follow the muscle groups involved in the lifts. If you don't work those muscles in reverse, they'll likely lose their plasticity over time, making it harder and hard for you to move. A good example is someone who does a lot of bench presses without performing compensatory movements. Their shoulders and chest get tighter and tighter and they tend to round forward and have bad posture and a weak upper back. They also start to get more injuries.

Compensatory movements can be stretches, but can also involve weights or bands. A compensatory movement for the bench press could be rows, whether with dumbbells, kettlebells or a rowing machine. The rowing action strengthens the upper back and helps the shoulders and chest maintain their correct alignments.

Do these as a sequence, holding each position for 3 to 5 breaths. The breaths should be slow and deep into the belly.

Cool-Downs

OVER UNDER

This stretches the lats, triceps and shoulders.

1 Stand tall. Take your right arm behind you and try to place the back of your hand on your left shoulder blade. Your palm will face away from your body. If you can't get your hand on the shoulder blade, you'll need to use a towel (see variation below). Reach your left arm up and over your left shoulder, palm facing toward your back, and try to hook the fingers of both hands together.

Repeat on the other side.

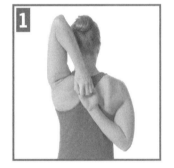

VARIATION: If you can't hook your fingers together, hold a towel in your high hand. Grab the towel in your low hand and walk the low hand up the towel as far as you can with minimal discomfort (remember, always 3 or less on the Rate of Perceived Discomfort scale). Pull up with the high hand, opening the low hand's shoulder, and hold for a 1 count. Pull down with the low hand to stretch the left triceps, holding for a 1 count. Repeat this 5 times each way.

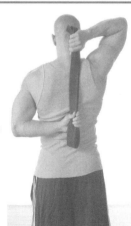

CHEST STRETCH

1 Stand tall, reach both arms behind you and interlace your fingers. Straighten your elbows if you can, stick your chest out and pull your shoulders back. If you can straighten your elbows, try to lift your arms a little higher behind you.

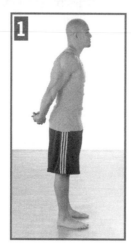

THORACIC STRETCH

I learned this stretch, referred to by some as the "Brettzel," from Gray Cook and Brett Jones.

- Lie on your left side, using a towel or pillow to support your head so that it's in a straight line with your spine and can stay relaxed throughout the stretch.

- Fold at your hips and knees and bring your hips as close to your chest as possible.

- Grab your right knee with your right hand and bring it in close to your chest.

- Take your left foot up behind you and try to get your thigh as far back as you can; grab your left ankle with your left hand.

- Rotate your upper body toward the right and try to place your right shoulder on the floor. Your neck should remain relaxed as you turn your head to the left to help with the shoulder rotation. Look over your shoulder with your eyes. Stay relaxed and breathe deeply, keeping your right knee up high to prevent low back issues and to maximize the benefit of this stretch.

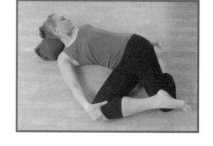

VARIATION: If you can't grab your rear ankle, use a towel or yoga strap.

UPWARD DOG

This classic yoga pose will help open the hip flexors and stretch the abs while strengthening the shoulders and triceps. This is an active pose; don't just hang out.

1 Lie on your stomach with your hands roughly beside your ribs and your fingers pointing forward; keep your elbows by your sides. Extend your legs behind you with the tops of your feet on the floor. Push the ground away, straightening your arms completely, so that only your palms and tops of your feet are on the floor. Reach your chest forward and up, keeping your shoulders down and away from your ears. Tilt your head back slightly, making sure not to crunch the back of your neck.

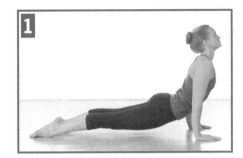

DOWNWARD DOG

Another classic yoga pose, this serves to stretch the shoulders, hamstrings, glutes and calves.

1 Start in high plank then drive your hips up and back, pushing back hard with your arms so that your head is between your arms but not hanging down; maintain a straight spine. From here, drive your heels toward the floor. You should feel a stretch in your calves and, if tight, your hamstrings and glutes. This, too, is an active pose so don't stay relaxed—push.

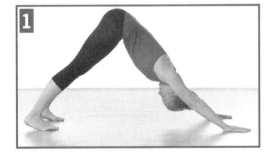

SLEEPING WARRIOR

1 Sit on the floor with your lower legs tucked under you and the tops of your feet flat on the floor. Bring your knees together as much as possible. Fold at the hips, reaching your butt to your heels, and extend your arms along the floor in front of you. Each time you exhale, sink your hips back and down, reach out more with your hands and think about elongating your spine.

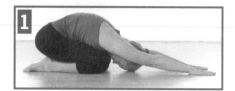

VARIATION 1: Push back with your arms instead of reaching out.

VARIATION 2: From the Sleeping Warrior position, rotate your elbows down and try to get your forearms on the floor. You should feel this in your lats as well as your lower back.

STRETCHING SEQUENCE

Here's a nice sequence that ties the Sleeping Warrior, Upward Dog and Downward Dog together.

1 Start in Sleeping Warrior and hold for 3 breaths.

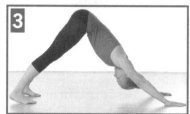

2 Stay low to the floor and extend your hips so your upper body moves through the arms until you're in low plank on your palms. Move into Upward Dog by pushing the floor away, lifting your torso, driving your shoulders down, sticking your chest out, arching your back and lifting your head. Hold for 3 breaths.

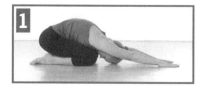

3 Move into Downward Dog by lifting your hips up and back, pushing hard with your hands and trying to get your heels to the floor. Hold for 3 breaths.

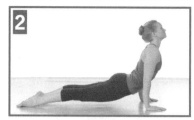

4 Bend your knees and flip your feet so the tops are on the floor and sink back into Sleeping Warrior. Do this sequence 3 to 5 times if time is short.

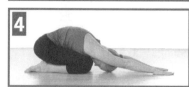

HAMSTRING STRETCH

This stretch loosens the hamstrings by raising the hips, not forcibly stretching them. It's a different effect than bending over and grabbing the feet.

1 Stand tall with your feet and knees together. Sink your hips down and back as far as you can and place your fingers under your heels. If you can't reach your heels, go to the sides of your feet or toes. Keep your hips down.

2 Pull hard against your feet and lift your hips up high; keep pulling on your feet and lifting your hips. After 3 breaths, if you aren't able to fully straighten your knees, bend your hips slightly then lift them again. This should allow your legs to be straighter.

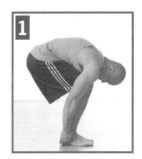

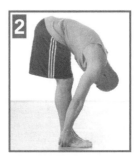

CAT/COW

The cat stretch opens the shoulder blades while the cow opens the abs and chest.

1 Place your hands and knees on the floor. Your hands are shoulder-width apart, right under your shoulders, and your knees are right under your hips so your thighs are vertical.

2 Tuck your pelvis under, exhaling as you do so. Suck your navel to your spine and push the floor hard with your arms. Lift your upper back and feel your shoulder blades move apart. Tuck your chin to your chest. Hold for 3 breaths.

3 Untuck your pelvis and chin at the same time, lifting both to the extreme opposite positions. Your hips are up, your low back is curved down and your head is up. Continue to drive the ground away with your arms. You should feel your abs being stretched. Hold for 3 breaths and move back to cat.

Repeat 3 times.

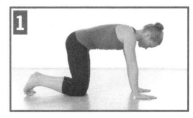

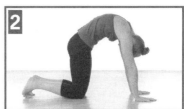

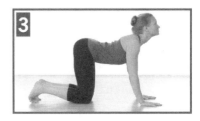

KNEES TO CHEST

This releases the lower back and is similar to Sleeping Warrior.

1 Lie on your back and bring both knees tightly to your chest. Wrap your arms around your shins and, if possible, grab your elbow with the opposite hand. If you can't wrap your arms around, hold your shins with your hands. As you exhale, pull your knees in more tightly.

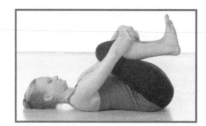

SEATED TWIST

Sit on the floor with both legs straight out in front of you. Place your right foot on the floor outside your left leg. Make sure both butt cheeks are on the floor throughout the stretch. Take your left arm across your right knee and rotate toward the right, moving from your waist first, then shoulders, then head. Press your left arm against your right knee and make sure you're sitting up tall. You should feel a stretch in your right hip, the piriformis muscle. The toes on your left foot point straight up.

Hold this for 5 breaths, slowly unwind and switch sides.

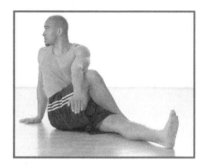

SAGE POSE

Sit on the floor with both legs straight out in front of you. Place your left foot on the floor outside your right leg. Tuck your right leg under your left hip, making sure your left buttock stays on the floor. Wrap around to the left and rotate as far as you can. Remember to stay tall.

Switch sides.

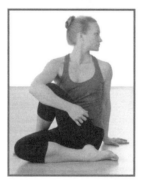

VARIATION: For an extra challenge, thread your right arm through your legs, bring your left hand around your back and try to bring your hands together.

SHOULDER BRIDGE

Also known as a hip extension or hip raise, this opens the hips as well as the lower and middle back. See page 61 for more details.

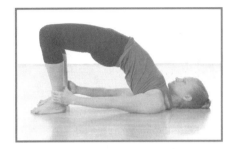

SHINBOX

If sitting in shinbox causes a discomfort level of 3 or more, stop immediately.

1 Sit on the floor and bend your left leg so your shin is parallel to your torso and your left foot rests against your right thigh just above the knee. Bend your right leg so your inner thigh is on the floor and your foot is by your right butt cheek. Try to keep both butt cheeks on the floor and stay tall.

2 Keeping your feet in place, lift both knees up at the same time. Due to lack of lower back mobility and/or weak abs, you may need to put one or both hands on the floor to keep from falling.

3 Flip both legs to the opposite side to sit in shinbox again (reverse view shown).

If your hips are tight, the shinbox will feel uncomfortable; use your hands to take some of the weight off your lower body. To switch sides, straighten both legs and reverse your position.

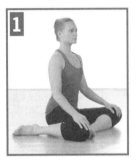
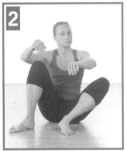
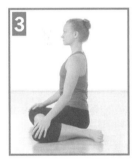

ADVANCED VARIATION: You can also work on opening your hips from shinbox by rising up onto your shins, using your hands if necessary to push yourself up. Once up on both shins, push your hips forward, squeeze your glutes and stick your chest out. Hold this for one breath, slowly sink back to shinbox position, flip your legs over and rise up on the other side.

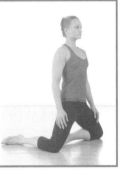

FOREARM STRETCH 1

1 Kneel on the floor and place one hand on the floor with the palm facing forward. Place the other hand on the floor for support if you wish.

2 Slowly roll the hand forward so that it's flat on the floor; try to keep your fingers pointing straight back but don't hyperextend your elbow. If you're unable to keep your fingers pointing straight back, rotate your forearm outward a little so that your fingers point to the outside of your leg. Take your time and feel the stretch in your fingers, palm, wrist and forearm.

Slowly returning to the starting position. Do 3 to 5 reps on each arm.

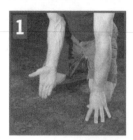

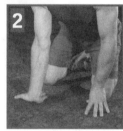

FOREARM STRETCH 2

1 Press your palms together in front of you, fingers up and forearms parallel to the floor.

2 Rotate your forearms so your fingers point forward.

3 Rotate your forearms until your fingers point at or touch your sternum. Your forearms should be close to parallel to the floor. Move your fingers away from your sternum by straightening your elbows while trying to keep your palms together. Once they've separated, bend your elbows and return to the starting position.

4–5 Keeping your palms together, use the fingers of one hand to push back the fingers of the other, trying to keep your fingers straight.

Push the other way then repeat the cycle 3 to 5 times.

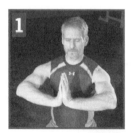

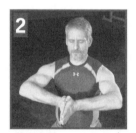

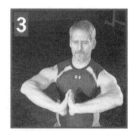

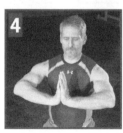

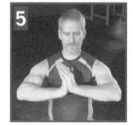

Pre-Hab

Whether you exercise hard or not, have a labor-intensive job or sit at a computer all day, pre-hab work will keep you from developing issues due to repetitive stress or the stresses placed on the body through lifting weights. Pre-hab work is meant to be preventive maintenance of the body.

While most of these movements can be done as a warm-up or cool-down, the focus here is on preventing injuries. It's not warming up or stretching out—it's movement or bodywork designed to correct alignment, break up muscles that are "stuck together," break up scar tissue…all of which are meant to help prevent injuries, as opposed to rehab, which fixes you after you're broken.

Please take the time to perform these pre-hab movements and see a massage therapist regularly. Your body will thank you. When you do pre-hab, you should be able to exercise harder with less discomfort, or maybe even no discomfort, and your recovery should occur faster. Best of all your chance of injury should go down as well.

JOINT MOBILITY DRILLS

Joint mobility drills can and should be done as pre-hab as well as part of your warm-up; they cross the boundary, as do many movements. The movements can be done anytime and most can be done anywhere. For desk-bound individuals, they're a great way to break up tension and recharge the body and mind. For everyone else, doing them throughout the day is a great way to take a break from work.

For example, doing the neck mobility series as described in the Warm-up section (pages 123–25) is a great way to loosen up the neck and reset the muscles in the upper back and chest. Sitting at a desk all day like most of us do creates poor posture, shortens the chest muscles (pectoralis major and minor) and weakens and overstretches the trapezius, rhomboids, levators and other muscles of the upper back. The result is a rounded upper back and protruding head—not a good thing. Practicing the neck series helps reset the muscles and the vertebrae; in addition, you should make sure you choose exercises that strengthen the upper back muscles (such as rows) and stay away from those that cause tightening of the upper torso (e.g., bench presses).

Self-myofascial release (sMFR) is a form of self-massage that uses a foam roller, tennis ball or golf ball to apply pressure to affected areas in order to get the muscles and fascia (connective tissue that surrounds all muscles and organs in the body) to relax. There are also specialized sticks that do the same thing. sMFR can be rather painful because it breaks up fibers that are stuck together and tend to be rather sensitive. Performing sMFR on a daily basis will help prevent problems from arising and help fix issues that may already be affecting your movement.

Fascia is intertwined with everything inside you. Because of this, everything you do affects more than just one area. If you lift your arms overhead, you'll feel your abdomen tighten. This is due to the fascia pulling the various abdominal muscles. Not only do the abs get pulled, the pelvis can get tipped, too, especially if your hips are tight. All muscles are connected to each other via the fascia and when any type of trauma occurs, even a minor incident like hitting the side of your leg, the fascia in that area tends to become restricted. This can cause pain in that area but can also cause pain in other areas of the body, many times on the opposite side. Pain away from the affected area, known as referred pain, can be difficult to pinpoint. You may not remember getting hit in the side of your leg but your knee or calf may ache for days.

If you've ever twisted an ankle, you've probably walked differently, maybe even limped, for a few days. What you may not have realized is that this throws your hips as well as your shoulders out of alignment; you may have started experiencing neck issues. If your ankle took a long time to heal, your body may have adapted to the new alignments in your body and you may be stuck with the new alignments even though your ankle eventually healed. If that's the case, you'll need sMFR or massage therapy as well as stretching and some strengthening to get the muscles and skeletal structure aligned normally. sMFR and massage therapy will locate the source of the problem and resolve the superficial issues caused by the injury or strain.

sMFR works via the slow application of pressure to a restricted area; this basically lets the restrictions "melt" away, separating fibers. When restrictions are caused by an injury, such as getting hit, or from undergoing surgery, it may only take one treatment to achieve full release of the restrictive area. In the case of restrictions caused by lots of intense exercise or severe trauma, you'll probably need to perform sMFR daily.

To perform sMFR, you'll need a foam roller, a tennis ball and possibly a golf ball. The foam roller, which can be purchased online and in some brick-and-mortar stores (sporting goods, Pilates, physical therapy), varies in length and diameter, up to about 4 inches in diameter and 3 feet long, down to 2 inches by 2 feet. Use a small roller for small areas, larger roller for larger areas. A tennis or golf ball is used for pinpoint rolling. There is also a tool called the "Stick," which is used to hit hard-to-get-to areas. You can get one at PerformBetter.com or other fitness supply websites or stores.

Typically the lower back, sides of the legs, quadriceps and hamstrings are rolled with a foam roller, and the glutes are usually worked by sitting on a tennis ball. The upper back can use a roller or either ball.

MASSAGE THERAPY

Massage therapy is also pre-hab. If you train hard, you need to have a good massage therapist help you release the built-up tension and trigger points that inevitably occur from not only heavy, hard training, but from everyday life. A good therapist can identify problem areas you may not even realize you have and then release or reduce the problem; you'll wonder how you ever functioned before. Most states license massage therapy so you should check with a potential therapist to see if he/she is state or nationally certified and how many hours of class time and clinical he/she did prior to becoming licensed.

SMFR: FOAM ROLLER AND SIDE OF THE LEG

1-2 Lower the side of your hip on the roller with your legs straight out, feet facing to the side. Support yourself with the arm on the side you're rolling and use that arm to pull your body so that your leg moves over the roller and back. This can be very painful in most people so you may want to place the other hand on the floor to help reduce the amount of pressure on your leg. Move slowly, stay relaxed and breathe. You don't want to cause more tension—you want it to go away. When the pain goes away (this may take many treatments), the trigger points and stuck tissue have been broken up (or perhaps you simply passed out from the pain). Do both sides.

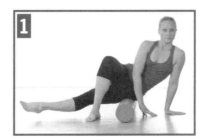

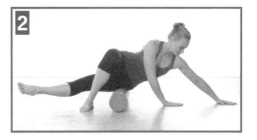

SMFR: FOAM ROLLER AND QUADS

1-2 Lie face down with one or both quads on the roller and place both hands on the floor. Use your arms to pull your body so that your thighs move up and down the roller. It's going to hurt, so go slowly, ease into it and breathe.

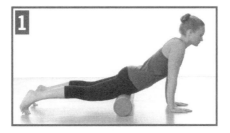

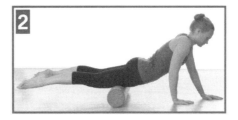

SMFR: FOAM ROLLER AND HAMSTRINGS

1–2 Sit on the roller, starting where your hamstrings meet your glutes; place your hands on the floor behind you. Just like the others, use your arms to move your legs up and down the roller.

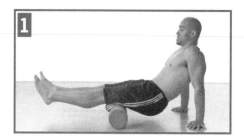

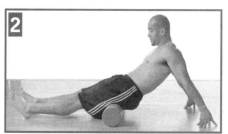

To roll other body parts, follow the same general guidelines. Place the body part on the roller and use your arms to move the body, adjusting the amount of pressure by raising or lowering your hips. When doing the inner thigh, go slowly and ease into it; it's a very sensitive area.

SMFR: BALL AND GLUTES

1 Sit on a tennis ball, adjusting the pressure by using your hands to lift you off the ball. Move your body around, gently applying pressure to the trigger point with the ball until it relaxes.

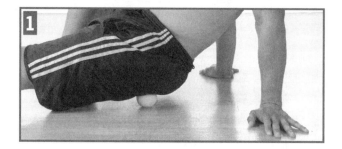

SMFR: BALL AND SHOULDERS

1–2 Lie face up with the ball under the affected shoulder. Move your body around on the ball, and adjust the pressure by using your legs to lift your hips.

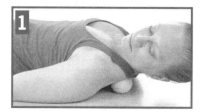

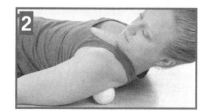

Resources

www.dragondoor.com   The source of many great products, including top-of-the-line kettlebells and Pavel Tsatsouline's *Enter the Kettlebell! Secret Strength of the Soviet Supermen* and *The Russian Kettlebell Challenge*

www.ikff.net   Features several excellent kettlebell and bodyweight DVD sets by Steve Cotter

www.rmaxinternational.com   The home of Scott Sonnon's joint mobility, Prasara Yoga, clubbell and bodyweight systems

Mark Rippetoe and Lon Kilgore's *Starting Strength* (Aasgaard Company, 2007) is great for beginner weightlifters; DVD available

Dr. Mel Siff's *Supertraining* (Verkhoshansky.com, 2009) and its facts and fallacies of fitness is a must-read for the serious trainee or trainer

Jamie Hale's *Knowledge and Nonsense: The Science of Nutrition and Exercise* (www.maxcondition.com)

Index

Other Ulysses Press Books

Black Belt Krav Maga: Elite Techniques of the World's Most Powerful Combat System

Darren Levine & Ryan Hoover, $15.95

As the official defensive tactics system of Israeli police, military and elite special operations units, Krav Maga has proven its effectiveness. For the first time, *Black Belt Krav Maga* teaches and illustrates the discipline's most lethal fighting and self-defense moves in book format.

Complete Krav Maga: The Ultimate Guide to Over 230 Self-Defense and Combative Techniques

Darren Levine & John Whitman, $21.95

Developed for the Israel military forces, Krav Maga is an easy-to-learn yet highly effective art of self-defense. Clearly written and extensively illustrated, *Complete Krav Maga* details every aspect of the system, including hand-to-hand combat moves and weapons defense techniques.

Corps Strength: A Marine Master Gunnery Sergeant's Program for Elite Fitness

MGySgt. Paul J. Roarke, $14.95

Renowned for its rigorous fitness training, the Marine Corps requires every member to be physically fit, regardless of age, grade or duty assignment. *Corps Strength* applies the same techniques used to develop and maintain each Marine's combat readiness to a day-to-day program for top-level fitness.

Dynamic Stretching: The Revolutionary New Warm-up Method to Improve Power, Performance and Range of Motion

Mark Kovacs, $14.95

Many top athletes and trainers have abandoned static stretching in favor of dynamic stretching. Now *Dynamic Stretching* teaches athletes and exercise enthusiasts everything they need to know about this breakthrough in sports performance.

Ellie Herman's Pilates Workbook on the Ball: Illustrated Step-by-Step Guide

Ellie Herman, $14.95

Combines the powerful slimming and shaping effects of Pilates with the low-impact, high-intensity workout of the ball.

Functional Training for Athletes at All Levels: Workouts for Agility, Speed and Power
James C. Radcliffe, $15.95

Teaches all athletes the functional training exercises that will produce the best results in their sport by mimicking the actual movements they utilize in that sport. With these unique programs, athletes can simultaneously improve posture, balance, stability and mobility.

Healthy Shoulder Handbook: 100 Exercises for Treating and Preventing Frozen Shoulder, Rotator Cuff and Other Common Injuries
Dr. Karl Knopf, $14.95

The step-by-step, self-healing program in this book offers a complete antidote to the most common shoulder problems.

Plyometrics for Athletes at All Levels: A Training Guide for Explosive Speed and Power
Neal Pire, $15.95

Provides the nonprofessional with an easy-to-understand explanation of why plyometrics works, the sports-training research behind it, and how to integrate plyometrics into an overall fitness program.

Total Heart Rate Training: Customize and Maximize Your Workout Using a Heart Rate Monitor
Joe Friel, $15.95

Shows anyone participating in aerobic sports, from novice to expert, how to increase the effectiveness of his or her workout by utilizing a heart rate monitor.

To order these books call 800-377-2542 or 510-601-8301, fax 510-601-8307, e-mail ulysses@ulyssespress.com, or write to Ulysses Press, P.O. Box 3440, Berkeley, CA 94703. All retail orders are shipped free of charge. California residents must include sales tax. Allow two to three weeks for delivery.

Acknowledgments

Big thanks to family and friends, who continually push me to learn and grow, encourage me to follow my dreams and give me the support to keep forging ahead. Especially (in no particular order): Lisa, Cheryl, Stephani, Julie, Paula, Jeanette, Marguerite and Paul. Also thanks to my kung fu instructor, Senior Master John Price, and the rest of my kung fu brothers and sisters.

Special thanks to Jamie Hale, who referred Ulysses Press to me when he was approached about writing this book and has given me guidance on several things since I've known him.

Pavel Tsatsouline, Steve Cotter, Scott Sonnon and the people in their respective organizations all have taught me a lot about kettlebells and training in general.

And thanks to Lily Chou and Claire Chun at Ulysses Press for the great work they did in editing and producing this book.

About the Author

Dave Randolph has been involved in martial arts since 1989, earning the rank of Associate Master, 5th-degree black belt, in 2005. Through his martial arts training and teaching, Dave became interested in teaching fitness to more than just martial artists. In 2002 he became a certified kettlebell instructor under Pavel Tsatsouline, who brought kettlebells into the mainstream around 1998.

Once certified (one of the first 100 certified by Pavel), Dave taught workshops to help bring kettlebells to the Louisville, Kentucky, area and taught kettlebell seminars in Atlanta and Cincinnati. Around the same time, he became a certified clubbell instructor under Scott Sonnon, and was one of the first 100 to be qualified to teach Sonnon's CST system. In 2007 Dave began teaching fitness full-time in Louisville's only full-time kettlebell-centric gym. During that time he became certified with several other top-level kettlebell instructors.

Dave's unique methods have helped thousands of people over the years become healthier and fitter. By integrating joint mobility, strength, agility, flexibility and coordination, Dave's IronBody Fitness shows people how to improve their lives. To contact Dave about teaching kettlebells in your area, visit his website www.iron-body.com or www.spartanwarriorworkout.com.